OXFORD MEDICAL PUBLICATIONS

Gynaecological Oncology

Gynaecological Oncology

A Guide to Clinical Management

Edited by

P. Blake
Consultant Clinical Oncologist,
The Royal Marsden NHS Trust, London

H. Lambert
Honorary Senior Lecturer/Honorary Consultant,
Hammersmith Hospital, London

R. Crawford
Gynaecological Oncology Fellow,
St Bartholomew's Hospital, London

OXFORD   NEW YORK   TOKYO
OXFORD UNIVERSITY PRESS
1998

Oxford University Press, Great Clarendon Street, Oxford OX2 6DP

Oxford   New York

Athens   Auckland   Bangkok   Bogota   Bombay
Buenos Aires   Calcutta   Cape Town   Dar es Salaam
Delhi   Florence   Hong Kong   Istanbul   Karachi
Kuala Lumpur   Madras   Madrid   Melbourne
Mexico City   Nairobi   Paris   Singapore
Taipei   Tokyo   Toronto   Warsaw

and associated companies in
Berlin   Ibadan

Oxford is a trade mark of Oxford University Press

Published in the United States
by Oxford University Press Inc., New York

A catalogue record for this book is available from the British Library

Library of Congress Cataloging in Publication Data

Gynaecological oncology: a guide to clinical management/edited by
P. Blake, H. Lambert, R. Crawford.
Includes bibliographical references and index.
1. Generative organs, Female—Cancer.   I. Blake, Peter R.
II. Lambert, Hannah E.   III. Crawford, R. (Robin)   IV. Series.
[DNLM: 1. Genital Neoplasms, Female—diagnosis.   2. Genital
Neoplasms, Female—therapy.   WP 145 G9975 1997]
RC280.G5G864   1997
616.99'465—dc21
DNLM/DLC
for Library of Congress   97–22258   CIP

ISBN 0 19 262798 8

Typeset by Footnote Graphics, Warminster, Wilts
Printed in Great Britain by
Bookcraft Ltd., Midsomer Norton, Avon

Preface

Gynaecological malignancy remains a major problem throughout the world with a different emphasis in developed and underdeveloped countries. Considerable progress is now being made in both areas and this progress extends from screening programmes to detect pre-invasive disease, to new surgical techniques for operable tumours and improvements in radiotherapy and chemotherapy for the treatment of advanced cancer.

The management of patients with gynaecological malignancy requires a multidisciplinary approach to include doctors, nurses, paramedics, and social workers, each of whom have their own expertise, and co-ordination between the various persons and teams involved, e.g. the primary care team, the treating hospital, hospice, and palliative care services, is paramount.

In order for the best care, treatment and advice to be given to the patient, a basic knowledge of gynaecological oncology is needed. The aim of this book, written by clinical oncologists, a gynaecological oncologist, a palliative care physician, and a specialist in gestational trophoblastic disease, is to provide that knowledge and includes guidance on the diagnosis, investigation, and treatment of the common gynaecological cancers and provide background information on the main treatment modalities. The book contains chapters dealing with gynaecological cancer at specific sites, namely the cervix, body of uterus, ovary, vulva and vagina, and gestational trophoblastic tumours. There is also a chapter on the molecular biology of gynaecological cancer, an area in which research might indicate how a susceptibility to these tumours may be inherited, and which might also give rise to novel treatments.

The latter half of the book provides information on the basic treatment modalities of surgery, radiotherapy, and chemotherapy as applied to gynaecological cancer. The book is completed by a chapter on palliative care, emphasizing the importance of an integrated multi-disciplinary approach to the patient throughout the course of her disease.

It is hoped that this book will be useful to trainees in oncology and gynaecology, both medical and nursing. In addition general practitioners, palliative care teams, and paramedical staff may find a guide to gynaecological oncology helpful in their work.

London   P.B.
September 1997   H.L.
                                                                                   R.C.

Contents

Contributors

H. Lambert *Honorary Consultant and Honorary Senior Lecturer in Clinical Oncology, The Hammersmith Hospital, London*

P. Blake *Consultant and Honorary Senior Lecturer in Clinical Oncology, The Royal Marsden Hospital, London*

R. Crawford *Lecturer, Gynaecology Oncology, St. Bartholomew's Hospital, London*

K. Broadley *Consultant in Palliative Care, The Royal Marsden Hospital, London*

E. Newlands *Professor in Medical Oncology, Charing Cross Hospital, London*

K. Harrington *Research Fellow, Clinical Oncology, IRCF, The Hammersmith Hospital, London*

Acknowledgements

A. Jeyarajah, Research Fellow in Gynaecological Oncology, St. Bartholomew's Hospital, London

I. Jacobs, Consultant Gynaecologist, St. Bartholomew's Hospital, London

K. McCarthy, Consultant Pathologist, Gloucestershire Royal Hospital, Gloucester

PART I

Gynaecological cancer at specific sites

1

Introduction

There are nearly 16 000 cases of invasive gynaecological cancer per annum in the United Kingdom. This accounts for over 20 percent of all cancers in women, although breast cancer remains the commonest female malignancy with around 25 000 cases per annum. The comparative incidence of cancers of the genital tract diagnosed in women in England and Wales, in 1988, is shown on Table 1.1. Against this background there has recently been an upsurge of interest in cancers of the female reproductive tract, leading to the development of specific screening programmes and new forms of therapy. Diagnostic clinics with immediate access to specialist expertise are also being developed.

Anatomy and staging

The female reproductive organs are situated in the pelvis and comprise the vulva, vagina, uterus, fallopian tubes, and ovaries. The anatomy of these structures and their relationship to the other pelvic organs is shown in Figs 1.1 and 1.2 and is given in detail in subsequent chapters.

Before a decision can be made about the therapy necessary for each patient the extent of the cancer must first be defined accurately. Disease spread is classified in such a way that not only reflects prognosis but which also allows a comparison of results of treatment to be made between departments world-wide. This classification is known as 'staging'.

Two main staging systems are used internationally in gynaecological cancer. The first is the TNM system of the UICC (International Union Against Cancer), which provides staging for tumours at any site in the body in terms of the primary tumour (T), lymph nodes (N), and metastases (M). The second system, which relates only to gynaecological cancer, is that of FIGO (International Federation of Gynaecology and Obstetrics) and this system is used throughout this book. The FIGO staging is identical to the T stage of the TNM system and is based on clinical, radiological, surgical, and histopathological findings. In general, the FIGO system requires less sophisticated imaging than the TNM system and is therefore applicable world-wide (UICC, 1992).

For all tumours the FIGO staging is divided into four main groups numbered I–IV. Stage I is the earliest stage with disease being confined to the organ of origin, and stage IV is the most advanced with other organs being

Table 1.1 Incidence of cancers of the genital tract diagnosed in women in England and Wales in 1988, by age (OPCS 1994)

Organ	Age <50 years (%)	Age >50 years (%)	No.	%
Ovary	16	84	5174	35
Cervix	44	56	4467	31
Endometrium	8	92	3789	26
Others	8	92	1125	8
Total			14 555	100%

OPCS, Office of Population Censuses and Surveys, London.

involved. Stages II and III describe intermediate degrees of spread. Within each stage there may be substages to describe the size, distribution, or grade of tumour.

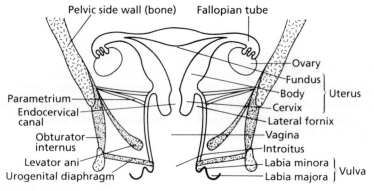

Fig. 1.1 Coronal view of the female pelvis showing the reproductive organs in relation to each other and to the pelvic side wall.

Pathology

The most common gynaecological tumours are epithelial in type, squamous carcinomas from the squamous epithelium of the cervix, vagina and vulva, and adenocarcinomas from the glandular tissue of the ovary and endometrium. Some organs, such as the ovary, contain several tissue types, epithelial, germ cell, and stromal, all of which can give rise to both benign and malignant tumours. Pathology, by confirming the diagnosis and establishing the extent of the disease, helps to determine the type of treatment that would be most appropriate in each patient. However, the flow of information between the clinicians and the pathologists must be two-way as the natural history of the disease, the findings at surgery, and the results of

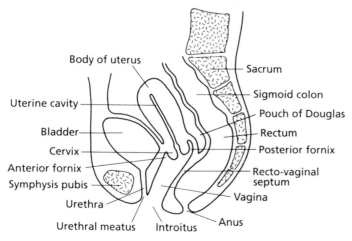

Fig. 1.2 Lateral view of the pelvic organs showing the relationship of the uterus and vagina to the bladder anteriorly and to the rectum posteriorly.

imaging investigations can provide valuable help to the pathologist who is otherwise making a diagnosis purely on the appearance of the tissue. It is important to hold pathology case conferences at which clinicians have the opportunity to view and discuss tumours with the pathologist.

Pathological diagnosis is usually made on tissue fixed in formalin which takes several days to process. However, fresh tissue can be examined within minutes of removal from the body if it is flash-frozen and sectioned immediately. Whilst the accuracy of diagnosis on frozen section is limited, it is a useful method of determining whether or not margins of excision during surgery are clear or whether lymph nodes are involved.

Special histochemical methods may help to resolve the precise diagnosis in some difficult groups of tumours, for instance uterine sarcomas, germ cell tumours and tumours that are anaplastic, or have no obvious cell of origin. Equally, staining of tissues with monoclonal antibodies may show the presence of tumour markers, such as carcino-embryonic antigen or CA125, that were not detectable in the patients serum, allowing a more specific diagnosis to be made.

The pathology of the common tumours in each of the gynaecological organs is discussed in detail in the specific chapters.

Treatment

Surgery

Surgery is the primary treatment for most gynaecological tumours and, in addition, plays a major part in diagnosis and staging. The surgical procedures involved may be of a local nature (e.g. the excision of a cervical cone in early microscopic cancer of the cervix), or very extensive, as in pelvic exenteration for recurrent cancer. All gynaecological cancer cases should be reviewed by a multi-disciplinary team and the surgery performed by an appropriately trained surgeon. In particular, radical hysterectomy and radical vulvectomy should be carried out by specialist-trained gynaecological oncologists.

Radiotherapy

Radiotherapy is the treatment of cancer by ionizing radiation which destroys the cancer cells whilst causing minimal damage to normal tissues. In patients with gynaecological tumours it may be used with curative intent or for palliation of a symptom. The radiation therapy is prescribed and supervised by clinical oncologists (known as 'radiation oncologists' outside the UK) and is delivered by therapy radiographers (technicians). Medical physicists and engineers are also needed to service the highly complex machinery needed to plan and deliver radiotherapy safely and correctly. As a consequence of the expenses of purchasing, installing, and running radio-therapy equipment, it is only available at cancer centres serving populations of 1–2 million people. In some areas this may mean that patients have considerable distances to travel for treatment.

Chemotherapy

Chemotherapy involves the use of drugs that interfere with the metabolism and replication of cells. If used correctly these drugs can have a more profound effect on malignant than normal cells and can lead to tumour shrinkage and, occasionally, cure. In gynaecological cancer chemotherapy is used in addition to surgery or radiotherapy except in the treatment of gestational trophoblastic tumours and the rare germ cell tumours, where it is the definitive treatment.

The drugs are usually given intravenously or, occasionally, orally and circulate systematically to treat the whole body. As these drugs can effect all cells they can produce severe side-effects and should be given under the supervision of specially trained oncologists. The administration of chemo-therapy, both as inpatient and as outpatient treatment is usually by specialist nurses. The pharmacist plays an important role in maintaining a register of treatment regimens and in checking the prescription against this to ensure that the correct drugs in the correct dosage are given to the patient with the necessary anti-emetics and other medications.

Performance status and treatment acceptability

Curative treatment for cancer, especially when in advanced stages, may be onerous and the patient must be fit enough to tolerate intensive therapy.

When a cure is not possible, therapy is aimed at improving the patient's well-being and must be well tolerated. To measure the effect of the disease and the impact of treatment on the patient an assessment of their general condition is needed. In addition this allows patient entry for therapeutic studies to be standardized and, therefore, several scales of performance status have been developed. One commonly used scale is the Eastern Cooperative Oncology Group (ECOG) scale (Table 10.5 p. 224).

All treatment has side-effects that can range from mild and temporary, such as nausea after chemotherapy, to severe and permanent, such as radiation bowel damage. In judging the acceptability of treatment, the goal of the therapy, either for cure or palliation, the side-effects and the performance status of the patient must all be considered. Ultimately, the patient must decide whether or not to proceed with treatment.

In order to do this, the patient must be fully informed by the multi-disciplinary team, of the likely consequences of treatment. Ideally, patient information should also be available in written form. This allows the patient and her carers to make a considered and unhurried choice. Information is now available for common tumours and treatments both on a local and national level with departmental information sheets and publications by organizations such as Cancer Link, BACUP (British Association of Cancer United Patients), and the Royal Marsden Hospital. Information sheets for patients entering clinical trials are a requirement of local research ethics committees. These can seldom answer all of a patient's questions because of the complex nature of clinical research, and the trial information sheet should be explained by a 'contact' person, such as a member of the research team.

Psychological problems, such as anxiety and depression, commonly arise. These may result from the diagnosis of cancer, which is often seen as leading inevitably to pain and death, from social and family implications of the disease, and from the treatment itself.

Hospitalization and travelling for prolonged outpatient therapy can add considerably to a patient's psychological and social problems. This can lead to a refusal to continue therapy. Supportive care is essential and should include both practical help with travel, expenses, and hostel arrangements and counselling by health workers.

Psychosexual aspects of gynaecological cancer

For a woman of any age the diagnosis of gynaecological cancer can be a crisis point. Support from her partner, medical and nursing staff at all stages of diagnosis, treatment and follow-up is important.

Sexuality is basic to how a patient 'sees herself' and makes a major contribution to her quality of life, both in a social and biological sense

(Andersen and van der Does 1994). If the relationship with her partner suffers then there may be disruption of the recovery process. Problems can be reduced by acknowledging sexuality as an area of discussion and providing support at an *early stage* in the clinician–patient contact. Information, which can be oral or written, or both, needs to be understandable and relevant. Despite both physical and psychological changes many women strive to remain sexually active. If there are sexual problems, counselling and advice on dealing with them should be given, if possible to both partners. Increasing awareness of the importance of dealing with the effect of gynaecological cancer on sexuality has resulted in increased training in this area particularly for specialist nurses. Hormone replacement therapy can also be helpful, and is suitable for most patients who have been found to have gynaecological cancer.

Fertility

Increasingly, the diagnosis of gynaecological and other cancers in young women does not need to lead to enforced sterility. Thirty-five years is the watershed below which there is a significant fertility rate, although there is still potential for childbirth at a later age. Certain gynaecological cancers, such as gestational trophoblastic disease and germ cell ovarian tumours, can be treated by chemotherapy without sterilization, and fertility can also be preserved by the use of limited surgery in superficial invasive cancer of the cervix and early stage epithelial cancer of the ovary.

Modern techniques of assisted conception are of little help for women treated for gynaecological cancer. At present, the most successful method is the freezing of embryos. This requires ovarian hyperstimulation prior to ovum harvest and subsequent fertilization, leading to a delay in the cancer treatment as well as possible harm to the patient from the high levels of oestrogens. Also, successful freezing of an embryo does not equate to a 'take-home' baby, even supposing a functioning uterus can be maintained following treatment or that a surrogate mother can be found. Cryopreservation of ovarian tissue is being offered although, to date, there have been no successful pregnancies from this technique.

The multi-disciplinary team

The multi-disciplinary approach to the management of the patient includes both primary care in the community and specialized hospital care. The latter should take place in a cancer centre or cancer unit and should extend beyond the specialist medical team of gynaecological, clinical and medical oncologists to include both general and specialist nurses, therapy radiographers, dietitians, and many others. This approach should be coordinated by an integrated care plan to aid communication between professionals, as well as with the patient. Regular gynaecological oncology unit meetings to discuss patients in a multi-disciplinary forum are also useful.

Central in this team is the patient's primary care physician or general practitioner (GP). Usually it is the GP who initially raises the possibility of the patient having cancer and who subsequently has to discuss the implications of hospital-based investigations and treatment with the patient and her family. Moreover, it is the GP who is in charge of the patient at home and who co-ordinates the domiciliary services, including hospice and community-based nurses. The GP will manage the patient's fears, pain and depression, possibly to a greater extent than the hospital specialist. Clear communication between the hospital and the GP is paramount. A frequent criticism made by GPs of hospital discharge summaries is that abbreviations (e.g. 'PMB' chemotherapy) and eponyms (e.g. 'Nigra' regimen) are used that are understood only within the specialist team. These terms should be avoided.

Palliative care specialists, both hospital and community-based, should be involved, preferably at an early stage, with those patients who have intractable symptoms or a limited life-span.

The interaction of medical staff caring for the gynaecological cancer patient is shown in Fig. 1.3 and the paramedical personnel involved in Table 1.2.

Table 1.2 Paramedical personnel involved in patient care

1. Nurses
   - Hospital-based
     – general
     – specialist (eg oncology, gynaecology, and stoma therapy)
   - Hospice-based (continuing care)
   - Macmillan (both continuing and home care)
   - District (home care)

2. Radiographers (therapy) and medical physicists

3. Social workers (hospital and community-based)

4. Others
   - Physiotherapist
   - Occupational therapist
   - Dietician
   - Pharmacist
   - Counsellors

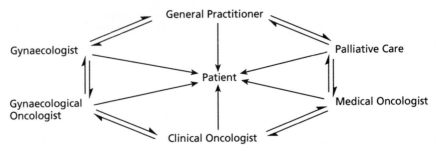

Fig. 1.3 The interaction of medical staff caring for the patient with gynaecological cancer.

Complementary medicine

Complementary therapies are increasingly being used in cancer care as more patients and their carers are interested in exploring all possible anti-cancer treatments. None of these complementary therapies have been the subject of critical review in randomized trials, but there is no doubt that they can give a patient a sense of confidence, hope, and of actively helping herself. The usual medical attitude is not to discourage patients from seeking complementary treatment so long as this is carried out in conjunction with normal medical practice.

However, caution is needed with special diets for therapy. Patients require balanced nutrition with all the necessary dietary elements. Some diets that are advocated to 'cure' cancer are neither palatable nor nutritionally sound and may be very expensive or difficult to obtain. In addition, many patients find that they cannot enjoy or even tolerate a diet that is completely different from their usual one and become frightened and depressed by their failure to comply with the new regime. High-fibre diets of raw foods may exacerbate symptoms due to radiation bowel damage or lead to obstruction if the bowel is involved by tumour, as may be the case with advanced carcinoma of the ovary.

Conclusions

The management of patients with gynaecological cancer is complex. It requires the combined expertise of hospital and community health professionals and good communication both between these workers and with the patient.

The aim of treatment is to cure the patient or to alleviate a symptom. This treatment should only be commenced after considering the likelihood of achieving that aim, the incidence and severity of side-effects, the performance status of the patient and full, informed discussion has taken place with the patient and her carers.

Reference

Anderson, B. L. and van der Does, J. (1994). Surviving gynecological cancer and coping with sexual morbidity: an international problem. *International Journal of Gynecological Cancer*, 4, 225–40.

UICC, International Union Against Cancer (1992). *TNM Atlas*. 3rd edition, 2nd revision. Eds. Spiessl, B. *et al*. Springer-Verlag, Berlin.

2

Cancer of the ovary and fallopian tube

CANCER OF THE OVARY

Incidence

Ovarian cancer is the most common gynaecological cancer in the United Kingdom, with 5174 cases being reported in 1988 (Office of Population Censuses and Surveys 1994). Most of these cancers are epithelial in origin. The lifetime risk of developing ovarian cancer is 1.5 percent which is considerably lower than the 7.1 percent lifetime risk of developing breast cancer. Ovarian cancer-related deaths per annum outnumber those from cancer of the cervix and endometrium combined. Most women present with advanced disease at diagnosis and 80–85 percent of such women will die of their disease. The overall survival for women with ovarian cancer is only 25–30 percent at 5 years.

Epithelial carcinomas of the ovary are rare before the age of 30 years and the incidence increases with age. Less than 20 percent of epithelial ovarian cancers are diagnosed before the age of 50 years and the peak incidence is in the 50- to 70-year-old age group. Germ cell tumours are found in children and young women, usually under 30 years of age.

Aetiology

The causes of epithelial ovarian cancer are not known. There is evidence that taking the contraceptive pill, which suppresses ovulation, reduces the likelihood of developing cancer of the ovary (Vessey *et al*. 1987). This fact, taken together with the knowledge that early menarche, late menopause, and nulliparity all increase the incidence, suggests that continuous ovulation may be an important aetiological factor.

Familial cancer

Inheritance plays a significant role in about 5 percent of epithelial ovarian cancers, usually serous adenocarcinomas. Families with multiple cases of ovarian cancer alone are rare, more commonly there are associated cases of breast, colorectal, or endometrial cancer—the Lynch syndrome (Watson and Lynch 1992). Where families show an autosomal dominant inheritance of breast and ovarian cancer, this is usually due to the presence of mutations in the BRCA1 gene. The presence of one of these mutations gives a lifetime risk of more than 30 percent for ovarian cancer. Mutations in a second gene BRCA2, discovered at the end of 1995, gives a lower risk in regard to ovarian cancer. In the general population the carrier frequency of BRCA1 mutations is approximately 1 in 800. This means that BRCA1 accounts for 3 percent of ovarian cancers below the age of 70 years and 6 percent of ovarian cancer below the age of 30 years (Yates 1996).

Genetic screening

BRCA1 mutation screening may be useful in familial and early onset breast and ovarian cancer, but it will have little significance in screening the general population because there is no firm evidence to show that the BRCA1 gene mutation contributes to *sporadic* cancer of the ovary. Genetic screening is discussed further in Chapter 7 on molecular biology.

Management of women with a history of familial ovarian cancer

The management of women identified as being at high risk of developing familial ovarian cancer is not clear. None of the available screening tests is known to be effective. It is important that any woman, considered to be at risk, is referred to a genetic clinic for counselling, further investigation or prophylactic therapy (see Chapter 7, p. 148).

Anatomy

The structure and function of the ovary varies with age. It enlarges after the menarche and becomes atrophic after the menopause. The ovaries are two almond-shaped bodies, dull white in colour, measuring $2 \times 1.5 \times 1$ cm and are situated on either side of the pelvis, lying within the peritoneal cavity below the bifurcation of the common iliac arteries, anterior to the sacroiliac joints and close to the fallopian tubes.

Each ovary consists of a central medulla surrounded by a cortex, which is itself surrounded by a layer of germinal epithelium. Blood vessels, lymphatics, and nerves enter through the medulla by way of the broad ligament. The cortex is the functional part of the ovary and consists of a dense stroma, ovarian follicles, and corpora lutea. The outer coat of the cortex is dense and fibrous and is known as the tunica albuginea. This is continuous with the peritoneum of the mesovarium which attaches the ovary to the posterior layer of the broad ligament. The ovary is suspended from the uterine cornua by the ovarian ligament which runs inside the broad ligament to the mesovarium. The lateral pole of the ovary is supported by the infundibulo-

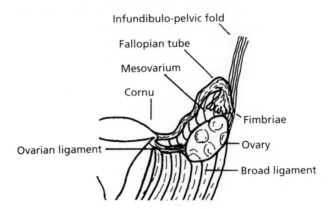

Fig. 2.1 Anatomy of the ovary (from the posterior aspect of the broad ligament).

pelvic ligament which contains the ovarian vessels and passes over the bifurcation of the iliac vessels on the pelvic side wall (Fig. 2.1). The ovary is related medially to the body of the uterus and the ovarian ligament and laterally to the infundibulopelvic ligament and the side wall of the pelvis. The broad ligament and the mesovarium lie anteriorly and the peritoneal cavity, the rectum, the sigmoid colon, and the sacroiliac joints lie posteriorly.

Lymphatic drainage

The lymphatic drainage is both to the pelvic and para-aortic nodes, the latter via the ovarian vessels. Lymphatic drainage is also to the sub-diaphragmatic lymphatic system, which drains the peritoneal cavity.

Spread of the disease

Cancer of the ovary invades the ovarian capsule and then spreads directly to involve the pelvic peritoneum and other pelvic organs. The peritoneal fluid carries malignant cells through the peritoneal cavity, to the omentum, to the peritoneal surface throughout the abdominal cavity including the peritoneal surfaces of the large and small bowel and liver, and to the surface of the diaphragm (Fig. 2.2). Metastases on the undersurface of the diaphragm may be found in over 40 percent of cases with disease apparently confined to the pelvis. Intraperitoneal metastases from ovarian cancer are characteristically superficial and seldom involve the substance of the underlying organ and even when the surface of the bowel is extensively involved, the muscularis layer is seldom infiltrated.

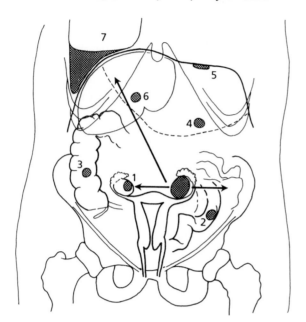

Fig. 2.2 Common sites of peritoneal involvement and routes of transperitoneal spread of ovarian cancer: (1) contralateral ovary and other pelvic organs; (2) loops of small bowel; (3) large bowel serosa; (4) omentum; (5) diaphragm; (6) liver capsule; (7) pleural cavity via diaphragmatic lymphatics.

Lymphatic spread

Lymphatic spread is mainly along the lymphatics that run with the ovarian vessels to the para-aortic region at the level of the renal vessels. These nodes may be involved in 15 percent of cases where the cancer is still within the pelvis (stages I and II) but involvement rises to 50 percent when the cancer has spread beyond the pelvis (stages III and IV). Pelvic lymph node involvement can be as high as for para-aortic nodes. Lymphatic spread may also involve the cervical and inguinal nodes. Malignant cells present in the peritoneal fluid may spread from lymphatic channels on the undersurface of the diaphragm to the pleura resulting in the formation of pleural effusions.

Blood-borne spread

Haematogenous spread usually occurs late with most women dying when the disease is still restricted to the peritoneal cavity. The main spread is to the liver and the lungs, although metastases to bone and brain are sometimes seen.

Pathology

There are a large number of different primary ovarian neoplasms. They are classified according to their tissue of origin into epithelial tumours, germ cell tumours, and sex cord stromal tumours. In addition, the ovary can be the site for lymphomas, sarcomas and metastatic disease. The tumours can be solid or cystic, benign or malignant or borderline. Borderline tumours are characterized by some of the cytological features of malignancy but lack any evidence of stromal invasion. A modified version of the World Health Organization (WHO) classification of ovarian tumours is shown in Table 2.1.

Epithelial tumours

Malignant epithelial tumours account for approximately 85 percent of ovarian cancers. They arise from the germinal epithelium of the ovary, which develops from the Mullerian duct, and is closely related to the cells lining the peritoneal cavity. The epithelium of most epithelial neoplasms resembles

Table 2.1 Modified histological classification of ovarian tumours (WHO)

 I. Common epithelial tumours (benign, borderline, and malignant)
  A. Serous
  B. Mucinous
  C. Endometrioid
  D. Clear cell (mesonephroid)
  E. Brenner
  F. Mixed epithelial
  G. Undifferentiated
  H. Unclassified.

 II. Sex cord stromal tumours
  A. Granulosa—theca cell tumour
  B. Sertoli–Leydig cell tumour
  C. Unclassified

 III. Germ cell
  A. Dysgerminoma
  B. Endodermal sinus tumour (yolk sac tumour)
  C. Embryonal carcinoma
  D. Choriocarcinoma
  E. Teratoma
  F. Mixed tumours

 IV. Soft tissue tumours not specific to ovary

 V. Unclassified tumours

 VI. Metastatic tumours

histologically that of parts of the urogenital tract of Mullerian origin, for example, *mucinous tumours* have epithelium resembling that of the endocervix, *endometrioid* that of the endometrium, and *serous* that of the endosalpinx (lining of the fallopian tube).

The commonest epithelial tumour is the serous adenocarcinoma, followed by the mucinous and endometrioid adenocarcinomas. There are also undifferentiated tumours which cannot be categorized and mixed tumours which show more than one type of epithelial cancer. Clear cell and Brenner tumours are rare.

Serous adenocarcinoma

These tumours, which are usually both solid and cystic, account for approximately 50 percent of all epithelial tumours. They are bilateral in about one-third of stage I cases (confined to the ovaries). Papillary patterns may be seen in the better differentiated tumours and psammoma bodies (calcospherites) are often present.

Mucinous adenocarcinoma

These tumours account for 10–15 percent of malignant ovarian tumours. They consist of multi-locular cysts containing mucinous fluid which can be huge, virtually filling the abdominal cavity. Macroscopically they may be mistaken for benign cysts and microscopically the more differentiated tumours will show tall 'picket fence' cells. Rupture of the capsule can give rise to *pseudomyxoma peritonei* in which a gelatinous material fills the peritoneal cavity. This condition can also be caused by benign or borderline mucinous tumours and by appendiceal mucocoeles.

Endometrioid adenocarcinoma

Between 10 and 15 percent of epithelial ovarian cancers are endometrioid tumours. They are frequently cystic, often unilocular, and contain brown fluid. The lining of the cyst usually has round polypoid projections and solid areas. Continuity with endometrioisis is seen in 5–10 percent of these tumours. As many as 15 percent of endometrioid carcinomas have concurrent cancer of the endometrium. Some of these tumours may be secondaries from one site to the other, but usually they appear to be two separate primary tumours.

Clear cell adenocarcinoma

These uncommon epithelial tumours, approximately 2 percent of the total, are usually unilateral. Microscopically they have a clear cell pattern, hence their name, and in some areas they show a tubular-cystic pattern with a 'hobnail' appearance of the lining epithelium. Because there is both an association between clear cell carcinomas and endometriosis and also because clear cell tumours frequently coexist with endometrioid carcinomas, it has been suggested that clear cell carcinomas may be a variant of endometrioid adenocarcinoma.

Grading

Malignant epithelial ovarian tumours are graded histologically into three groups: (a) well differentiated, *grade 1*; (b) moderately differentiated, *grade 2*; (c) and poorly differentiated, *grade 3*. Well-differentiated epithelial tumours of the ovary tend to be more often associated with early stage disease.

Borderline epithelial tumours

Ten per cent of epithelial ovarian tumours are borderline tumours. An alternative name for these tumours is 'epithelial tumours of low malignant potential'. The majority are serous or mucinous in type. These tumours show features of malignancy such as varying degrees of nuclear atypia and an increase in mitotic activity, multilayering of neoplastic cells, and formation of cellular buds, but unlike adenocarcinoma of the ovary, there is no invasion of the stroma (Ovarian Tumour Panel, RCOG, 1983).

Most borderline tumours remain confined to the ovaries but occasionally they present with peritoneal lesions some of which are metastases. However, many of these lesions are not true metastases, and they may remain stationary or even regress after removal of the ovarian primary (Fox 1985). The majority of borderline tumours are serous or mucinous and in the latter the diagnosis of borderline malignancy from early invasive disease can be particularly difficult. Other types of borderline tumours are rare.

Other malignant ovarian tumours

Metastatic carcinomas account for most of the ovarian tumours that are not epithelial in origin. The primary tumours that most commonly give rise to ovarian metastases are of the endometrium, breast, and gastrointestinal tract. Differentiation from primary ovarian cancer can be difficult, in advanced cases, particularly in the case of colonic tumours.

'Krukenberg tumour' is a term often used to describe secondaries to the ovary although true Krukenberg tumours, usually derived from a stomach cancer, have a distinct morphology, being solid kidney shaped tumours which microscopically contain mucin-secreting signet-ring calls.

Malignant sex cord and germ cell tumours are not common and sarcomas are very rare.

Clinical staging

The FIGO staging of ovarian cancer is shown on Table 2.2. This is a surgico-pathological staging. It includes cytological examination of ascites or peritoneal washings and is dependent on the findings at laparotomy in

Table 2.2 FIGO staging for primary ovarian carcinoma

Stage I	Growth limited to ovaries	
Ia	Growth limited to one ovary	No ascites; no tumour on external surface; capsule intact
Ib	Growth limited to both ovaries	No ascites; no tumour on external surface; capsule intact
Ic	Stage Ia or Ib	Ascites containing malignant cells; *or* with positive peritoneal washings; *or* tumour on external surface of one or both ovaries; *or* with capsule ruptured
Stage II	Growth involving one or both ovaries with pelvic extension	
IIa	Extension and/or metastases to the uterus or tubes	
IIb	Extension to other pelvic tissues	
IIc	Stage IIa or IIb	Ascites present containing malignant cells; *or* with positive peritoneal washings
Stage III	Growth involving one or both ovaries with peritoneal implants outside the pelvis; *or* positive retroperitoneal; *or* inguinal lymph nodes. Superficial liver metastases equals stage III	
IIIa	Tumour grossly limited to the true pelvis with negative nodes, but with histologically confirmed microscopic seeding of abdominal peritoneal surfaces	
IIIb	Tumour with histologically confirmed implants on abdominal peritoneal surfaces none exceeding 2 cm in diameter. Nodes are negative	
IIIc	Abdominal implants greater than 2 cm in diameter; *or* positive retroperitoneal; *or* inguinal nodes	
Stage IV	Growth involving one or both ovaries with distant metastases*	

FIGO, International Federation of Gynaecology and Obstetrics.
*If pleural effusion is present there must be positive cytology. *Parenchymal* liver metastases equals stage IV.

the majority of cases. Parenchymal involvement of the liver is necessary to make a patient stage IV, peritoneal deposits on the surface of the liver being included in stage III. If a pleural effusion contains malignant cells, it is also stage IV.

Diagnosis

Symptoms and signs

Symptoms

Approximately 70 percent of patients are diagnosed when the ovarian cancer has advanced beyond the ovaries (Table 2.3). This is due to the insidious nature of the symptoms and signs of carcinoma of the ovary but occasionally it is due to a rapidly growing tumour. Patients may complain of indigestion, vague abdominal discomfort, a feeling of pressure in the pelvis, urinary frequency, weight loss and, most frequently, swelling of the abdomen. Rarely, patients may complain of abnormal menses or post-menopausal bleeding. Due to the non-specific nature of most of these symptoms, the diagnosis of ovarian cancer is seldom considered at first presentation.

Signs

The presence of an abdominal mass arising from the pelvis, particularly in the presence of ascites, is highly suggestive or malignancy. A fixed, hard, irregular pelvic mass is felt best by combined vaginal and rectal examination. In very late cases supraclavicular or inguinal nodes may be palpable.

Investigations

It is crucial to the management of this tumour that the full extent of disease is defined before treatment. This will usually be made from the surgico-pathological findings at laparotomy. The investigations, prior to surgery, for ovarian cancer include a full blood count, serum biochemistry, tumour markers, X-rays, and other imaging techniques.

Table 2.3 Results of treatment for ovarian cancer by stage (modified from FIGO 1988)

Stage	% of total	% alive at 3 years	% alive at 5 years
I	26	80	73
II	15	60	46
III	39	27	19
IV	16	10	<5
Overall			25–30

Imaging techniques

Ultrasonography, both abdominal and transvaginal may help to confirm the presence of a pelvic mass and detect ascites before it is clinically apparent. An ovarian cancer typically presents as a semi-solid, semi-cystic mass with thick septae and surface papillations. In addition, ultrasound is a reliable technique for examining the hepatic parenchyma and may detect enlarged pelvic or para-aortic lymph nodes. Computed axial tomography (CT) can give similar information and is more likely to detect enlarge nodes but is more expensive and exposes the patient to radiation. Magnetic resonance imaging (MRI) is particularly useful for examining the pelvis.

None of these imaging techniques will image small peritoneal metastases which can be seen by the naked eye at laparotomy. *Laparotomy remains the most important investigative tool for the diagnosis and staging of ovarian cancer.*

Cytology

Cytological examination of pleural effusions or ascites can be carried out for the presence of malignant cells. Fine needle aspiration of clinically suspicious nodes in the neck or groin can be valuable in assessing disease spread.

Tumour markers

The most useful tumour marker in epithelial ovarian cancer is the antigen *CA125*, derived from a human cancer line. CA125 is a high molecular weight glycoprotein recognized by the antibody OC125. This is useful in the diagnosis of epithelial ovarian cancer but it is not specific enough or sensitive enough to establish the diagnosis on its own. Peritoneal irritation from endometriosis or pelvic inflammatory disease can lead to a raised level of CA125 and it can also be raised in other abdominal malignancies, if they are in an advanced stage.

The level of CA125 is elevated in over 90 percent of cases of advanced ovarian cancer (i.e. stages II–IV), but in only 50 percent of women with stage I disease (Jacobs 1995). By adding to CA125, one or more of a panel of tumour markers such as the human milk factor globulins 1 and 2 (HMFG1/2), placental alkaline phosphatase (PLAP), macrophage colony stimulating factor (M-CSF), or OVX1, the diagnostic sensitivity of the test can be improved.

Carcino-embryonic antigen (CEA) may be raised in mucinous cystadeno-carcinoma, concentrations in excess of 20 ng/ml being suggestive of ovarian tumour. *Inhibin* is another marker that has been found to be raised in mucinous tumours. Inhibin is also a useful marker in granulosa cell tumours.

Tumour markers for germ cell tumours should be measured if the woman is under 40 years of age. These tumour markers are alpha fetoprotein (αFP) and beta human chorionic gonadotrophin (βHCG), both produced by tumour elements. Lactic dehydrogenase (LDH) and PLAP may also be raised.

Screening for sporadic ovarian cancer

As already discussed, epithelial ovarian cancer is usually detected only when it is advanced, because of the lack of symptoms. A population screening test, which was able to detect ovarian cancer in its early stages, would be expected to reduce mortality. An ideal test would have both maximum *sensitivity*, that is the ability to detect all positive cases, and also complete *specificity*, in that it would be able to correctly identify all true negatives. The efforts to find such a screening test have been concentrated on using serum tumour markets and on ultrasonography of the ovaries. At present there are no genetic tests suitable for sporadic cancer.

CA125 for screening

As stated previously, CA125 is the most useful marker for ovarian cancer. However, it is not considered to be sufficiently specific or sensitive to be suitable, on its own, to screen the general population. Not only are CA125 levels frequently normal in stage I ovarian cancer, but in addition, CA125 has a lower specificity in premenopausal than in postmenopausal women, probably reflecting the raised levels of the tumour marker that can be obtained with menstruation and with benign disorders, such as endometriosis and pelvic inflammatory disease. Serial measurements of CA125 improve its specificity, as the levels rise in patients with preclinical ovarian cancer but remain static or fall in those with false positive results (Jacobs 1995).

The sensitivity of CA125 can be improved, without losing specificity, by either taking a lower cut-off point as a normal level, for example, 30 Units per ml (U/ml) rather than the accepted level of 35 U/ml, or by using additional tumour markers. Jacobs (1995) achieved a sensitivity of 80 percent and a specificity of 91 percent with the use of the two tumour markers CA125 (at a level greater than 25 U/ml) and OVX1 (at a level greater than 12 U/ml). Very raised levels of serum CA125 in asymptomatic postmenopausal women, 100 units or greater, indicate a high risk of ovarian cancer in the following year (Jacobs *et al.* 1996).

Ultrasonography for screening

Ultrasonography can detect enlargement and structural changes in the ovary. Conventional abdominal ultrasonography has not been found to be sufficiently accurate in detecting tumours in asymptomatic, postmenopausal women to be used as the sole screening investigation. The accuracy of ultrasonography has been improved by using transvaginal ultrasound with colour-flow Doppler, which not only gives a better view of the ovaries than an abdominal scan but also detects alterations in blood flow. This technique was assessed in 1601 high-risk women with a family history of ovarian cancer (Bourne *et al.* 1993). A laparotomy or laparoscopy was carried out in 61 women with an abnormal scan of whom six had ovarian cancer, five being stage Ia, and a further three patients had borderline tumours. Using transvaginal ultrasound and colour-flow Doppler, a new randomized trial is to be carried out by the European Randomized Trial of Ovarian Cancer Screening (ERTOCS). Women will be placed in one of three groups, a control group and two to be screened with vaginal ultrasonography at intervals of either 1.5 years or 3 years. Those found to have an increased volume of ovarian tissue or abnormal morphology will have a colour-flow Doppler examination and, if this is abnormal, surgery will be performed. Results will not be available for several years.

Combined approach

A large study of 22 000 postmenopausal volunteers was performed at the Royal London Hospital using both CA125 measurements and abdominal ultrasound in order to improve the specificity of screening. Yearly CA125 was the initial investigation, followed by an abdominal ultrasound scan in those women identified as having a raised CA125 level. Forty-nine cancers developed in the study population over a follow-up period of nearly seven years. The cumulative risk of developing ovarian cancer was appreciably raised for those women with a CA125 concentration of 30 units or more (Jacobs *et al.* 1996).

A new randomized trial has started at the Royal London Hospital which will involve postmenopausal women in a study group versus control group. The women in the study group will have annual CA125 and OVX1 tumour marker measurements. On the basis of these results and age-adjusted ovarian cancer incidence rates, a risk score of cancer (ROC) will be calculated for each woman. If the ROC exceeds the study threshold, vaginal ultrasonography will be performed as second-line screening. If this is abnormal, laparoscopy or laparotomy will be carried out. The study will have an 80 percent power to detect a 30 percent reduction in mortality in the screened group compared to the control group who do not undergo screening (Jacobs 1995).

Screening: conclusions

In our present state of knowledge, and with the available technology, screening the general population to reduce the mortality from ovarian cancer is not of proven value. The results of randomized trials are awaited but this will take several years. Cost and acceptance of the procedure, as well as accuracy are important factors in devising any screening test.

Treatment of epithelial ovarian cancer

Both surgery and chemotherapy have major roles in the treatment of ovarian cancer. Surgery is the initial treatment both for accurate diagnosis, staging and therapy. Post-operative (adjuvant) chemotherapy is usually given, except for some early cases, where disease is confined to the ovaries, which are treated with surgery alone. Radiotherapy is mainly used for palliation.

Surgery

Laparotomy is essential for both staging and treating ovarian cancer. A satisfactory exposure is necessary in order to explore the whole abdomen adequately and, therefore, a vertical incision is better than a transverse incision. A sample of ascitic fluid or peritoneal washings, for cytological evaluation, is taken first. Following this, a systematic examination of the omentum, subdiaphragmatic areas, anterior abdominal wall, paracolic gutters, surface of the small and large bowel, pelvic organs, and pelvic and para-aortic nodes is made. Biopsies of suspicious areas are taken in the absence of gross upper abdominal disease. Using an Ayre's spatula, a subdiaphragmatic scrape may be taken to check for microscopic peritoneal involvement.

Primary surgery

Primary surgery is performed at or near the time of diagnosis. The aim of primary surgery is to remove all tumour. This is known as *cytoreductive or debulking surgery*. Although this is possible in early cancer of the ovary (i.e. stage Ia and Ib), it becomes less achievable as the tumour becomes more advanced and spreads throughout the abdominal cavity. The surgery for ovarian epithelial cancer is hysterectomy, bilateral salpingo-oophorectomy and infracolic omentectomy plus the removal, if feasible, of tumour masses outside these organs. The infracolic omentum is removed, even when it is not apparently involved, because it is a common site for microscopic disease. In early disease, in order to complete surgical staging, some surgeons perform a pelvic and para-aortic lymphadenectomy but this is not general practice in the UK at present.

Over the past 20 years, maximum cytoreductive surgery has been advocated on the premise that women with minimal residual disease (i.e. <1–1.5 cm in diameter) or with no residual disease after surgery, have a better prognosis than those in whom bulkier disease remained. However, the effect of debulking surgery in improving prognosis in advanced disease is not proven and it may well be that those patients, in whom complete debulking is possible, have a tumour that behaves in a different biological manner from those that cannot be debulked. In addition, patients with large metastatic disease (>10 cm diameter) or ascites at presentation, have a poor median survival whatever the amount of cytoreductive surgery. Other surgical indicators of a poor prognosis include carcinomatosis, extensive mesenteric involvement, and the performance of bowel surgery. Bowel surgery should not be carried out unless obstruction is imminent. Radical lymphadenectomy and the removal of all tiny tumour nodules, in advanced disease, is not recommended as there is no evidence that this improves outcome.

Whatever the effect of cytoreduction on outcome there is no doubt that cytoreduction improves the quality of life for patients and renders them more able to withstand subsequent chemotherapy. Cytoreductive surgery should always be attempted, and is successful in up to 75 percent of cases.

Interval (intervention) debulking surgery

Interval, or intervention, debulking surgery is the term used for a planned procedure performed in advanced ovarian cancer, when primary surgery is incomplete and has been followed by several courses of chemotherapy. Following surgery, chemotherapy is continued.

The effect of interval debulking surgery has been assessed by a randomized EORTCS study comparing chemotherapy alone with chemotherapy and interval debulking surgery in advanced ovarian cancer (Van der Berg *et al.* 1995). This study demonstrated that median survival may be extended by 6 months and survival at three years increased by up to 20 percent in the group undergoing the additional surgery.

Conservative surgery

Young women with a borderline or good prognosis early stage ovarian cancer, stage Ia well or moderately differentiated epithelial tumours, who wish to have a family, can be treated with a unilateral salpingo-oophorectomy alone. As there is some doubt about the safety of conservative surgery, it is paramount that a good staging procedure is first performed to exclude occult advanced disease. This would include endometrial sampling as the uterus is left *in situ*. The removal of the other ovary is advisable following completion of the patient's family as the rate of recurrence or new tumour formation in the remaining ovary is unknown.

Secondary surgery

Secondary surgery includes second look surgery, secondary debulking, and palliative surgery.

Second look surgery refers to laparoscopy and laparotomy performed to assess the effect of chemotherapy in patients who appear to have had a complete clinical and radiological response. Laparotomy is more accurate than laparoscopy and allows excision of residual disease but there is no evidence that second look surgery affects outcome and it is therefore of no clinical benefit.

Secondary debulking surgery should only be carried out as a planned procedure as for interval surgery. It has seldom been found to be of value in patients who have completed a course of chemotherapy and who still have persistent disease.

Palliative surgery is most often carried out for bowel obstruction. It should be avoided when the obstruction is in the small bowel as multiple areas are usually involved and the symptoms are frequently due to interference by the tumour with neuromuscular transmission.

Post-operative treatment

Except for good prognosis early stage ovarian cancer, chemotherapy is given following surgery, as not all microscopic disease will have been removed, however extensive the operation.

Stage I

In stage I, where tumour is confined to the ovaries, there is a need to define those cases at risk of recurrent disease and therefore requiring post-operative treatment. FIGO stage Ic includes capsular penetration by tumour, rupture of the capsule, malignant ascites or positive peritoneal washings, but there is little evidence that each of these has the same prognostic significance. Dembo (1992) found that poor differentiation of the tumour, large volume of ascites, and positive peritoneal washings were poor prognostic factors in stage I disease. Similarly, Vergote *et al.* (1993) found that the most important prognostic signs in stage I disease were poor differentiation of tumour, aneuploidy, and substage. Rupture of the capsule during surgery has not been found to be significant but, when occurring prior to surgery, it indicates a poorer prognosis (Sjovall *et al.* 1994).

There have been few randomized trials of post-operative therapy in stage I ovarian cancer, but in one of these, the Gynecologic Oncology Group (GOG) found a survival rate of over 90 percent in patients with low to intermediate grade tumours confined to the ovaries, regardless of whether or not they received adjuvant single agent chemotherapy (Young *et al.* 1990).

These data suggest that patients with stage Ia or Ib well or moderately differentiated tumours may be treated by surgery alone but that all other cases require adjuvant therapy. The International Collaborative Ovarian

Table 2.4 Current ICON randomized ovarian cancer studies

Study	Starting date	Randomization
ICON 1 Early stage ovarian cancer (Chemotherapy not clearly indicated)	1991	Treatment deferred until indicated *vs* Immediate platinum-based chemotherapy
ICON 2 Advanced ovarian cancer (Chemotherapy clearly indicated)	1991	CAP *vs* carboplatin
ICON 3 Advanced ovarian cancer	1995	CAP or carboplatin *vs* Paclitaxel and carboplatin
ICON 4 Relapsed ovarian cancer (Previously treated with chemotherapy and therapy free interval >6 months)	1996	Platinum-based chemotherapy *vs* Paclitaxel and a platinum drug

ICON, International Collaborative Ovarian Neoplasm Group; CAP, cisplatin, doxorubicin, and cyclophosphamide

Neoplasm Group (ICON 1) are comparing, in early cancer of the ovary, immediate adjuvant platinum therapy with treatment deferred until recurrent disease is detected (Table 2.4). The findings of this trial should help in further identifying the role of adjuvant therapy in early stage ovarian cancer.

Radiotherapy

Radiotherapy is little used in the modern management of ovarian cancer where it has been superseded by the development of more active chemotherapy. Whole abdominal radiotherapy had been found to lead to increased survival in early stage disease, when compared with pelvic radiotherapy plus the cytotoxic drug chlorambucil (Dembo *et al.* 1979). This work by Dembo remains important in that it emphasized that the whole abdominal cavity was at risk of occult metastases and therefore needed treatment. The total dose delivered to the whole abdomen, by external irradiation, was limited in order to protect radiosensitive organs such as the liver and kidneys. This limitation of dose resulted in external radiotherapy being ineffective for treating residual ovarian disease, unless it was microscopic.

Following chemotherapy, whole abdominal radiotherapy has been compared to further chemotherapy, as *consolidation* therapy in patients with advanced ovarian cancer found to have no or minimal disease at second look surgery. No advantage was found for consolidation radio-therapy compared to chemotherapy, even in those patients with no residual disease at second look surgery (Lambert *et al.* 1993).

It is therefore concluded that, at present, there is no role for external radiotherapy in ovarian cancer as part of a *radical* course of treatment. Radiotherapy is, however, useful for palliation, for example, to relieve pressure symptoms in the pelvis, vaginal bleeding, or metastatic deposits in the brain or bone.

Intraperitoneal radiotherapy

Radioactive isotopes of gold [^{198}Au] or phosphorus [^{32}P], linked to colloidal carriers, have been used intraperitoneally for many years in early carcinoma of the ovary, either alone or in combination with external radiotherapy. Radioactive phosphorus is used in preference to gold because 10 percent of the activity of ^{198}Au is gamma radiation, which is a hazard to both patients and staff.

Radioactive isotopes act by being absorbed on to the peritoneum where they are taken up by macrophages. Only the superficial 4–6 mm of peritoneal lining receives a high dose of radiation and most of the dose received by intra-abdominal organs is from the isotope absorbed into the circulation.

Trials in women with no residual tumour after primary surgery, comparing radioactive phosphorus to chemotherapy, have not demonstrated an advantage to either mode of treatment in regard to both disease-free survival or overall survival. One trial, comparing six courses of cisplatin with ^{32}P in nearly 350 patients without residual disease after primary surgery found no difference in disease-free or overall survival but a high incidence of late bowel complications in the phosphorus group (Vergote *et al.* 1992). There are no studies comparing intraperitoneal radioactive phosphorus with no treatment in early stage disease to discover whether there is any survival benefit. Studies, using both external and intraperitoneal radiotherapy, have found the combination caused a high incidence of severe bowel problems and this regimen is therefore not recommended.

A different approach using intraperitoneal radioimmunotherapy is with yttrium-90 attached to monoclonal antibodies such as human milk factor globulin 1 (HMFG 1). This experimental technique looks promising as consolidation therapy in women in apparent pathological remission after surgery and first-line chemotherapy (Hird *et al.* 1993), and a randomized trial of no further treatment versus intraperitoneal therapy is in progress.

Chemotherapy

Chemotherapy plays a central role in treating epithelial ovarian cancer. Except for patients with stage Ia and Ib well or moderately differentiated tumours, adjuvant chemotherapy is given after surgery and occasionally as primary treatment before interval debulking surgery. There has been an evolution of chemotherapy for ovarian cancer since the treatment was first introduced in the 1950s. (For more information, see Chapter 10 on chemotherapy.)

Alkylating drugs (excluding platinum drugs)

Historically, the chemotherapeutic agents most commonly used in carcinoma of the ovary have been the alkylating agents that were used initially as palliative treatment but later as adjuvant therapy, after surgical debulking became standard primary treatment. Initial response rates of 35–65 percent, were reported but were maintained in only 5–15 percent of patients after two years. The main drugs used were melphalan, chlorambucil, and cyclophosphamide. Later, ifosfamide and treosulphan, both alkylating agents, came into use.

Initial regimens were usually based on a single agent, for example chlorambucil or melphalan, but more complex regimens using multi-drug combinations became popular which included other drugs that showed some activity in treating ovarian cancer. These included the antimetabolites, 5-fluorouracil (5FU) and methotrexate, the cytotoxic antibiotics (e.g. doxorubicin), and the oral aziridine alkylating agent, hexamethylmelamine. The most active of these regimens was HexaCAF (hexamethylmelamine, cyclophosphamide, methotrexate, and 5FU) (Young *et al.* 1978). This multi-agent regimen was thought to improve survival rates compared to the single alkylating agent, melphalan. However, a meta-analysis, carried out by the Advanced Ovarian Cancer Trialists Group (AOCTG) analysing data from over 3000 patients in 16 randomized trials, found no advantage for non-cisplatin combinations over a single alkylating agent.

Alkylating agents remain important in the management of ovarian cancer. Chlorambucil is used for elderly patients and cyclophosphamide is commonly used in combination regimens. Ifosfamide and treosulfan are also useful agents. Hexamethylmelamine, which can be given by mouth, is mainly used as second-line treatment in relapsed patients.

Platinum drugs

The platinum drugs are the most widely used drugs in the management of ovarian cancer either alone or in combination. They are heavy metal compounds which cause cross linkage of the DNA strands in a similar fashion to alkylating drugs. Cisplatin was first used in the 1970s for patients who had failed alkylating agents. Response rates of 30 percent were obtained which led to its use as first-line chemotherapy.

There is no clear evidence to show whether or not platinum alone, or in combination, is superior to the alkylating drugs. A comparison of cisplatin with cyclophosphamide, as first-line chemotherapy in advanced ovarian cancer, showed a statistically significant advantage for cisplatin (Lambert and Berry 1985), but the AOCTG study comparing single or combination non-platinum regimens with the same regimens plus a platinum drug, was unable to show a survival advantage in favour of platinum. The explanation for this is thought to be, in part, due to platinum drugs being used as salvage therapy for patients relapsing from alkylating therapy, therefore the overview has, in effect, examined immediate versus delayed platinum therapy and failed to show a difference.

Despite the lack of clear-cut survival data, platinum-based therapy has been adopted as the standard therapy against which new regimens must be judged. This is partly due to the fact that clinical response is consistently greater with platinum therapy (approximately 75 percent), thus improving quality of life for patients.

Two platinum drugs are in common use at the present time, cisplatin and carboplatin. Cisplatin causes severe nausea and vomiting but this is usually well controlled with $5HT_3$ receptor antagonists such as ondansetron and granisetron. Cisplatin can give rise to severe renal damage, unless it is given with a forced diuresis and to peripheral neuropathy, which can last for several months. The latter appears to be dose-related. Cisplatin can also cause some high-tone hearing loss and hypomagnesaemia but it is not particularly myelotoxic.

The cisplatin analogue, carboplatin, has significantly fewer complications than cisplatin with almost no renal or neurotoxicity but it does cause nausea and vomiting and is marrow-toxic. Its efficacy has been compared with cisplatin in several studies. The overview by AOCTG (1991) confirmed that in over 2000 patients in 11 randomized trials there was no significant difference in survival between cisplatin and carboplatin. As carboplatin does not require hydration, it can be given on an outpatient basis.

Cisplatin is given in a dose of 75–100 mg/m^2 but the dose of carboplatin is calculated according to the AUC (area under the curve) Calvert *et al.* formula (1989), which is based on the glomerular filtration rate derived from EDTA clearance, or by using the Cockcroft formula (see Chapter 10, p. 211). This allows a higher dose of carboplatin to be given in the presence of normal kidney function as the myelotoxicity of carboplatin is related to renal function. The current recommended dose for chemotherapy-naïve patients uses an AUC factor of 5–9.

Single vs combination platinum chemotherapy   There is an issue of whether platinum as a single agent is equivalent to platinum in combination in terms of survival. The AOCTG overview was unable to reach a firm conclusion but their analysis suggested that platinum combinations were better than single-agent platinum at the same dosage. This led to the establishment of an international study to try to resolve this issue. The ICON 2 study compares cisplatin, doxorubicin, and cyclophosphamide (CAP) in combination, with single-agent carboplatin (see Table 2.4). The inclusion of doxorubicin in the combination is based on an overview analysis suggesting an 8 percent survival advantage for patients receiving doxorubicin in addition to cyclophosphamide and cisplatin (Ovarian Cancer Meta-analysis Project 1991). Interim results, presented in 1997, failed to show a *significant* survival difference between single-agent carboplatin and the platinum combination. The final result is awaited.

Taxane drugs

The taxanes are a new class of compounds that act by stabilizing microtubules in the cell, blocking division and thus tumour growth. They are active in ovarian cancer. Paclitaxel has been found to be the most active drug ever tested in patients with platinum-resistant ovarian cancer. In addition to myelosuppression and sensory neuropathy these drugs have an unusual toxicity profile including hypersensitivity reactions (up to 2 percent of patients, despite premedication). Hair loss is usually total, irrespective of dose, but nausea and vomiting are mild in contrast to the platinum drugs. The dose schedule varies between Europe and the USA. In Europe, 175 mg/m^2 is given over 3 hours whereas in the USA only 135 mg/m^2 is given but this is spread over a 24-hour period. Both schedules have been found to be equally effective.

A major trial carried out by the Gynecological Oncology Group (GOG, McGuire *et al.* 1996), randomized approximately 400 women with advanced ovarian cancer and residual disease of over 1 cm after initial surgery, to receive cisplatin plus either paclitaxel or cyclophosphamide. Surgically verified complete response was similar in the two groups, but median survival and progression-free survival were significantly better in the cisplatin–paclitaxel group, being 38 versus 24 months and 18 versus 13 months, respectively. The effect on longer-term survival is as yet unknown. On the basis of this study cisplatin–paclitaxel combination is now accepted as the standard therapy for advanced ovarian cancer in the USA.

There is little to suggest that paclitaxel as a single agent is superior to the platinum drugs and more studies are under way to ascertain its precise role in the management of ovarian cancer. The EORTC is conducting a similar trial to the GOG trial discussed above and ICON-3 is randomizing patients between carboplatin (or CAP) given 3-weekly for 6 courses and carboplatin plus paclitaxel, 3-weekly for 6 courses (see Table 2.4). Such comparisons are essential if the most active regimens with the least toxicity are to be used for large populations on a cost-effective basis.

Docetaxol (Taxotere) is a semi-synthetic taxane and early studies indicate that it has similar activity to paclitaxel but has an unusual skin toxicity and can produce marked oedema.

Other new drugs

New agents that are under investigation in patients with ovarian cancer include gemcitabine, a pyrimidine antimetabolite which has been found to be active in patients with platinum-resistant disease, and the topoisomerase I inhibitor, Topotecan, which is also active in platinum-resistant disease (see Chapter 10, p. 218).

Experimental chemotherapy studies to improve survival in advanced ovarian cancer

Despite the evidence that modern chemotherapy has improved median survival for advanced ovarian cancer (stages III and IV) from 12–18 months to 2–3 years, survival at 5 years remains poor, being 25–30 percent overall (see Table 2.3). This is true even for those patients who had a complete pathological response to surgery and chemotherapy. Many methods to improve the salvage rate have been tried. These have included high dose chemotherapy, intraperitoneal therapy, altering drug scheduling, and reducing drug resistance.

The effect of high dose chemotherapy has been studied with the platinum drugs but no survival benefit compared to standard therapy has been found so far. This may be because dose intensity needs to be seven to ten times higher than standard dose if drug resistance is to be overcome and current studies are unable to achieve this level of dose intensification.

Intraperitoneal therapy is an attractive method for treating ovarian cancer because the natural history of the disease is of extensive local peritoneal implantation without more widespread metastatic disease. While this route of therapy exploits the difference between intraperitoneal and absorbed intravenous concentrations, it is only suitable for treating small superficial deposits because the penetration of the drug is limited. However, this approach, using cisplatin, has been tested in a randomized study by Alberts *et al.* (1996) against intravenous cisplatin in patients with stage III cancer of the ovary and residual tumour deposits of 2 cm or less. This study found both improved median survival and lower toxicity for the intraperitoneal route (see Chapter 10, p. 219).

The above approaches and drug resistance are discussed further in Chapter 10 on chemotherapy.

Treatment of relapsed epithelial ovarian cancer

Cure of relapsed patients is not a realistic goal and, therefore, therapy is given with palliative intent and quality of life must be the first consideration. Some prolongation of survival may occur if second responses are obtained.

At present, treatment for relapse is usually offered when the patient is symptomatic. It is not known whether there is any benefit in early detection and treatment prior to the onset of symptoms. The tumour marker CA125 has been found to be useful in monitoring response to chemotherapy, a persistent rise may precede clinical evidence of recurrent disease by several months. A current Medical Research Council study is addressing this problem. It is comparing immediate second-line treatment in asymptomatic women on the basis of raised CA125 measurements greater than twice the upper limit of normal, with treatment deferred until clinically indicated.

Repetition of a platinum chemotherapy regimen will give responses if at least 6 months has elapsed between the end of initial chemotherapy and evidence of recurrent disease. The longer the interval between initial chemotherapy and relapse the greater the chance of a second response and the longer the survival (Gore 1990).

The taxanes, hexamethylmelamine, topetecan, and gemcitabine all show responses in platinum-resistant disease. A new trial by the ICON group (ICON 4) is concerned with patients with relapsed ovarian cancer previously treated with chemotherapy and having a therapy-free interval of greater than 6 months. Patients are randomzied to receive platinum-based chemotherapy with or without paclitaxel (see Table 2.4). This is to see whether the combination of a platinum drug with paclitaxel, with their differing modes of action on the tumour cell, is more effective than the platinum regimen alone. No dose reduction is required as both cisplatin and carboplatin can be safely combined with paclitaxel.

Other treatments used in relapsed ovarian disease include hormonal therapy, discussed below, and radiotherapy which may reduce symptomatic tumour masses. New approaches are also under investigation, for instance the use of Marimastat which inhibits matrix metalloproteinases, enzymes that promote spread and dissemination of solid tumours, including ovarian cancer.

Hormonal therapy

Cytoplasmic oestrogen and progesterone receptors have been detected in malignant ovarian tumours. However, the use of progestogens in recurrent disease has been disappointing, except for giving a feeling of well-being. Tamoxifen, at a dose of 40–80 mg daily, occasionally causes some partial response or stabilization of disease and the GnRH analogues, goserelin and buserelin, given subcutaneously every month, have also been reported as showing antitumour activity in patients with progressive disease.

Hormone replacement therapy

Hormone replacement therapy (HRT) in premenopausal women treated for ovarian cancer probably does not adversely affect the prognosis. A retrospective study assessed nearly 400 young women given HRT following treatment for ovarian cancer and showed no detrimental effect on prognosis (Eeles *et al.* 1991).

Immunotherapy

Immunotherapy has been used for carcinoma of the ovary for many years but is of unproven benefit. Non-specific immunotherapy with BCG (Bacille Calmette–Guérin) or *Corynebacterium parvum* has been combined with chemotherapy and appeared to prolong response. More recently, subcutaneous alpha-interferon has been the focus of interest and is being assessed, following chemotherapy, by the Yorkshire Ovarian Group to evaluate its role in prolonging overall and disease-free survival. Intraperitoneal immunotherapy with alpha-interferon for residual disease following initial chemotherapy has also been investigated and has resulted in some complete responses.

Prognostic factors and results

Borderline tumours

Although most patients with borderline tumours have a very good prognosis, there is a small group where the prognosis is poor. Prognosis appears to be mainly related to ploidy, with patients with aneuploid tumours having a 19-fold risk of death from disease compared to patients with diploid tumour (Kaern *et al.* 1993). Increasing age, stage greater than I, and non-serous histology are additional poor prognostic factors.

The overall 5-year survival for serous borderline epithelial tumours is 90–95 percent at 5 years and 60–85 percent at 15 years. The survival at 5 years for stage I borderline tumours is nearly 100 percent but drops to 65–85 percent for stage III disease. The longer-term prognosis is less certain.

Invasive tumours

The prognostic factors affecting long-term survival in epithelial adenocarcinomas of the ovary have been identified in several studies. They include stage, size of residual tumour after primary surgery, and performance status as, for example, measured by the Eastern Cooperative Oncology Group (ECOG) criteria (Table 2.5). DNA ploidy and overexpression of some oncogenes are also indicators of survival.

The effect of stage can be seen from the 5-year survival figures shown on Table 2.3. While stage Ia and Ib tumours with well or moderately differentiated histology have a 5-year survival rate of over 90 per cent, other early ovarian tumours have a worse prognosis, particularly if they are poorly differentiated and aneuploid. Ploidy is also an important prognostic factor

Table 2.5 ECOG Performance status

Grade	Performance status
0	Able to carry out all normal activity without restriction
1	Restricted in physically strenuous activity but ambulatory and able to carry out light work
2	Ambulatory and capable of all self-care but unable to carry out any work: up and about more than 50% of waking hours
3	Capable of only limited self-care: confined to bed or chair more than 50% of waking hours
4	Completely disabled: cannot carry out any self-care: totally confined to bed or chair

ECOG, Eastern Cooperative Oncology Group.

with patients having diploid tumours surviving significantly longer than those with aneuploid tumours.

In advanced tumours, as previously discussed, patients with large volume disease at the outset have a poor prognosis even after successful cyto-reduction. However, the extent of residual tumour after surgery appears to be the most highly significant prognostic factor in advanced ovarian adeno-carcinoma. No residual disease has the best prognosis and >2 cm has a poor prognosis.

Table 2.6 Prognostic factors affecting long-term survival

Variable	Multivariate analysis (P)
Residual disease microscopic to >5 cm (after initial surgery)	0.0004
Grade of tumour (ECOG)	0.013
Performance status (FIGO)	0.05
Stages Ic–IV	n.s.
Age	n.s

P, probability; n.s., not significant.
Table modified from Gadduci *et al.* (1996)

Gadduci *et al.* (1996), followed up 131 patients with stages Ic–IV treated between 1982 and 1994. The most important independent prognostic factors were found to be residual disease after initial surgery, performance status as measured by ECOG criteria and grade of tumour (Table 2.6). Age is a less important prognostic sign but women over 70 years have a poorer prog-nosis. *Angiogenesis*, the development of new vessels by the tumour, is also related to prognosis with denser microvessel involvement being associated with a poor prognosis.

Oncogenes as prognostic indicators

HER-*2/neu (c-erb B-2)*, an oncogene that codes for an epidermal growth factor (EGF) receptor protein, is overexpressed in about 30 percent of ovarian cancers (Berchuck *et al.* 1990). This overexpression of the EGF receptor was found to be the most sensitive indicator of a poor prognosis when the value of different oncogenes as prognostic indicators in ovarian tumours was studied by Van Dam *et al.* (1993).

p53 Gene mutations are found in up to half of the women who have advanced ovarian cancer (Marks *et al.* 1991). There is a lower incidence of mutations in early stage disease suggesting that the occurrence of mutated *p53* is a late event in the development of ovarian cancer. Alternatively, such mutations may result in rapid progression of disease. (Further information, see Chapter 7, p. 142).

Non-epithelial tumours

Non-epithelial tumours account for 10 percent of all ovarian tumours, the most common being the germ cell tumours and the sex cord stromal tumours.

Germ cell tumours

The most commonly occurring germ cell tumour is the *dysgerminoma*. Germinal epithelium contains primitive cells that have the potential to develop into both embryonic and extra-embryonic tissue—the placenta and the membranes. These cells are known as *totipotent* cells and can themselves give rise to tumours—*the embryonal carcinomas*—or they can develop some way along the normal pathway to embryonic or extra-embryonic tissues before becoming malignant, forming the *teratoma* from embryonic cells and the highly malignant *endodermal sinus tumour* and *choriocarcinoma* from extra-embryonic cells. Their derivation from germ cells is shown in Fig. 2.3 (Teilum 1965).

Germ cell tumours occur in young women. They are rare but it is important to recognize them at surgery so that conservative surgery is carried out to retain fertility. Chemotherapy is the main treatment modality and can cure many of these patients without compromising their chances of future pregnancies. Radical surgery, such as bilateral oophorectomy, does not improve cure rates.

Investigations, as well as including those for suspected epithelial ovarian cancer, such as chest X-ray and CT scan, should also include the examination of serum for the tumour markers alpha-fetoprotein (αFP) produced by yolk sac cells and the beta-subunit of human chorionic gonadotrophic (βHCG) produced by syncytiotrophoblastic elements of the tumour (Table

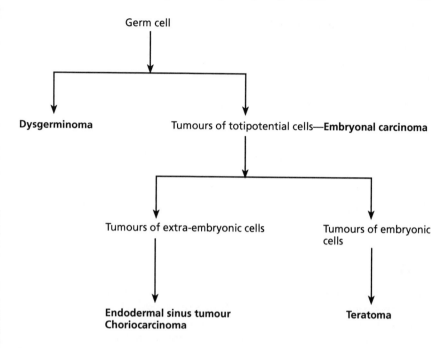

Fig. 2.3 Derivation of germ cell tumours. (From Teilum 1965.)

Table 2.7 Production of αFP and βHCG tumour markers by germ cell tumours

	αFP	βHCG
Dysgerminoma	–	rare
Embryonal carcinoma	+/–	+/–
Endodermal sinus tumour	+	–
Choriocarcinoma	–	+
Teratoma (immature)	+/–	–
Teratoma (mature)	–	–

αFP, alpha-fetoprotein; βHCG, human chorionic gonadotrophin.

2.7). Lactate dehydrogenase (LDH) and placental alkaline phosphatase (PLAP) should also be estimated.

Dysgerminomas

Dysgerminomas account for 2–5 percent of all primary malignant ovarian tumours and 40 percent of malignant germ cell tumours. They occur in women less than 30 years old. They behave in a similar fashion to seminoma in men, spreading by lymphatics to para-aortic, mediastinal and supra-clavicular glands. The serum tumour markers αFP and βHCG should normally not be raised but should always be assessed to rule out a mixed tumour with teratomatous elements. Occasionally, some cases of pure dysgerminoma do have raised levels of βHCG, and in metastatic disease PLAP and LDH are usually elevated.

Macroscopically, dysgerminomas are soft, rubbery solid tumours with a smith or nodular outer surface. They can grow to a large size. Microscopically they characteristically have large round cells separated by fibrous tissue septae infiltrated by lymphocytes. The tumour is bilateral in 10–15 percent of cases.

Treatment is by surgery. If, after staging, disease is found to be confined to one ovary, a unilateral oophorectomy with biopsy of the contralateral ovary is sufficient treatment. Even with bilateral tumours every effort should be made to maintain some normal ovary to preserve hormone production and fertility.

Pure dysgerminomas, like seminomas, are very radiosensitive and require only low doses of radiation but chemotherapy is both effective and does not lead to the inevitable ablation of the ovaries caused by radiation. Mixed dysgerminomas contain other malignant elements and unlike pure dysger-minomas, are not radiosensitive. Chemotherapy is therefore necessary for these tumours. The chemotherapy regimens are discussed below.

Pure dysgerminomas have a good prognosis as the majority, 75 percent, are stage I tumours and are usually stage Ia.

Other germ cell tumours

These tumours, like dysgerminomas occur in young women. Usually only one ovary is involved. Historically, malignant germ cell tumours had a very poor prognosis but this has been greatly improved by the use of combination chemotherapy.

Mature teratomas behave in a benign fashion. The most common is the cystic teratoma or *dermoid cyst* found at all ages. Dermoid cysts can contain many mature tissues including thyroid, teeth, and cartilage. Immature teratomas may contain areas of pale pink, immature neural tissue. Microscopically, rosettes of neuroectodermal cells with dark nuclei are the most conspicuous feature of these tumours.

Endodermal sinus tumours are the second most common malignant germ cell tumour of the ovary, after dysgerminomas, comprising 10–15 percent of the total. They are usually solid and areas of necrosis or haemorrhage may be present. Microscopically, the tumour consists of a loose vacuolated network of microcysts lined by flat cells. The most characteristic feature is the endodermal sinus (Schiller–Duval) body.

The tumour markers αFP and βHCG, when present, are valuable in diagnosis, monitoring therapy and in the follow-up of patients to detect early recurrence. Embryonal carcinomas can produce both proteins, whereas endodermal sinus tumours only produce αFP and choriocarcinomas βHCG (see Table 2.7).

Treatment The definitive treatment is chemotherapy, surgery being conservative with the aim of establishing the diagnosis, removing the primary, and staging the disease. Initial surgery in young women with *any* tumour affecting only one ovary should be unilateral oophorectomy as further surgery, if necessary, can always be carried out at a later date, once the diagnosis has been confirmed histologically.

Combination chemotherapy is given to all patients except for stage I malignant teratomas. The latter may be followed up at regular intervals with clinical examination, serum tumour markers, and radiological review, as the majority will not relapse and delayed treatment will not compromise survival. Chemotherapy is with cisplatin in combination, usually with bleomycin and etoposide (BEP). This is curative in the majority of patients with germ cell tumours who do not have adverse features such as very high levels of tumour markers, very bulky disease or involvement of the liver of central nervous system. A short but intensive course of chemotherapy, POMB/ACE, is an intensive regimen given over a short period (Newlands and Bagshaw 1987). This regimen alternates cisplatin, vincristine, methotrexate, and bleomycin with actinomycin-D, cyclophosphamide, and etoposide every two weeks for three to five courses. This regimen does not interfere with fertility and there have been no congenital abnormalities reported in children born to mothers who have received this chemotherapy.

Sex cord stromal tumours

Granulosa and theca cell tumours

Granulosa and theca cell tumours are the most common sex cord stromal tumours accounting for 1.5 percent of all malignant ovarian tumours. They are also the largest group of functioning ovarian tumours producing steroid hormones, mainly oestrogens, which can cause bleeding in older women and precocious puberty in girls. These tumours can occur at any age but are most frequent in postmenopausal women. The effect of the oestrogens produced by the tumour can result in endometrial hyperplasia or endometrial cancer. Inhibin can be used as a tumour marker for granulosa cell tumours. Pure theca tumours, which are usually benign, are virtually unknown. Most tumours are a mixture of benign theca and malignant granulosa elements. Macroscopically, these tumours are solid or cystic and the cut surface is often yellow because of the high lipid content. Microscopically, the most characteristic pattern is microfollicular, in which tumour cells are arranged in large groups in which are many Call–Exner bodies, small rounded cavities containing eosinophilic material.

Staging is the same as for epithelial tumours. Most, 85 percent, present as stage Ia with bilateral tumours only being present in 5 percent of cases.

Sertoli–Leydig cell tumours

These are very rare tumours, half of which produce male hormones causing virilization. Rarely, oestrogens are secreted.

Treatment for sex-cord stromal tumours   Surgery is the main treatment and is the same as for epithelial tumours (i.e. is bilateral salpingo-oophorectomy, hysterectomy, and infracolic omentectomy. Unilateral oophorectomy is indicated only in young women with stage Ia disease to preserve fertility. Granulosa cell tumours can recur many years after the initial diagnosis and in cases of late recurrence repeat surgery should be considered before any other therapy is given. The effect of adjuvant therapy is difficult to assess because of this tendency to recur late. Granulosa cells are considered to be moderately radiosensitive but it is more usual to treat advanced and early recurrent disease with chemotherapy, using the same regimens as for epithelial ovarian adenocarcinomas. The overall 5-year survival is around 80 percent, but advanced stage and recurrence is associated with a high mortality.

Conclusions: epithelial and non-epithelial tumours

The 5-year survival rate for epithelial cancer of the ovary is 25–30 percent (Fig. 2.3). It has changed little over the last 20 years. Only those cancers which are well or moderately differentiated and are confined to the ovaries have a good prognosis.

Most ovarian cancer presents when the disease is advanced. Effective screening of the general population to detect borderline tumours or early cancer is not possible at present. Treatment is by surgery followed by chemotherapy usually with a platinum-based regimen. Newer drugs, particularly the taxanes, give promise for improved disease-free survival in the future but at present survival depends more on the biological factors inherent in each tumour than on treatment. Despite side-effects, modern cytotoxic therapy has improved the quality of life for many patients.

Germ cell tumours which occur in young women have a much better prognosis than the common epithelial cancers. Treatment is primarily by chemotherapy which is not only curative but also preserves fertility.

CANCER OF THE FALLOPIAN TUBE

Primary carcinoma of the fallopian tube is very rare comprising 0.3 percent of all gynaecological malignancies. Most tumours involving the fallopian tube are metastatic from ovarian cancer but secondary spread from the breast and gastrointestinal tract can also occur. Cancer of the fallopian tube occurs after the menopause and is usually unilateral. Tumour spread is identical to that of ovarian cancer and metastases to pelvic and para-aortic nodes are common.

Pathology

The similarity in histology between serous adenocarcinoma of the ovary and primary tubal carcinoma means that strict criteria must be applied before the diagnosis of primary tubal carcinoma can be made. These criteria are that, on gross examination the main tumour is in the tube, microscopically the mucosa is chiefly involved and has a papillary pattern and, if the tubal wall is involved to a great extent, the transition between benign and malignant tubal epithelium can be demonstrated. The tumour usually distends the lumen of the tube and may protrude through the fimbrial end and the tube may be retort shaped, resembling a hydrosalpinx. Microscopically, the histological pattern is papillary with a gradation from alveolar to solid as the degree of differention decreases.

Staging

Surgical findings are the basis for the clinical staging for fallopian tube cancer and staging is similar to that of the ovary.

Diagnosis

Most cases of carcinoma of the fallopian tube are diagnosed at laparotomy. The diagnosis is seldom considered pre-operatively. The usual presenting symptom is postmenopausal bleeding and there may also be watery discharge and lower abdominal pain. Unexplained postmenopausal bleeding or abnormal cytology without an obvious cause may be due to cancer of the fallopian tube and bimanual examination and ultrasound should be carried out under such circumstances.

Treatment

The treatment for cancer of the fallopian tube is surgical and is the same as for cancer of the ovary. Post-operative platinum based chemotherapy is required for all but the earliest cases.

Results

The overall 5-year survival rate is around 35 percent but is in the region of 70 percent if the tumour is diagnosed while still confined to the fallopian tube.

References

Advanced Ovarian Cancer Trialists Group (1991). Chemotherapy in advanced ovarian cancer: an overview of randomised clinical trials. *British Medical Journal*, **303**, 884–93.

Alberts, D. S., Liu, P. Y., Hannigan, E. V. *et al.* (1996). Intraperitoneal cisplatin plus intravenous cyclophosphamide versus intravenous cisplatin plus intravenous cyclophosphamide for Stage III ovarian cancer. *New England Journal of Medicine*, **335**, 1950–5.

Berchuck, A., Kamel, A., Whitaker, R. *et al.* (1990). Overexpression of HER-2/neu is associated with poor survival in advanced ovarian cancer. *Cancer Research*, **50**, 4087–91.

Bourne, T. H., Cambell, S., Reynolds, K. M. *et al.* (1993). Screening for early familial ovarian cancer with transvaginal ultrasonography and colour blood flow imaging. *British Medical Journal*, **306**, 1025–9.

Calvert, A. H., Newell, D. R., Gumbrell, S. *et al.* (1989). Carboplatin dosage: Prospective evaluation of a simple formula based on renal function. *Journal of Clinical Oncology*, **7**, 1748–56.

Dembo, A. J. (1992). Epithelial ovarian cancer: the role of radiotherapy. *International Journal of Radiation, Oncology, Biology, Physics*, **22**, 835–45.

Dembo, A. J., Bush, R. S., Beale, F. A. *et al.* (1979). The Princess Margaret Hospital Study of ovarian cancer: Stated I, II and asymptomatic III presentations. *Cancer Treatment Report*, **63**, 249–54.

Eeles, R. A., Tan, S., Wiltshaw, E. *et al.* (1991). Hormone replacement therapy and survival after surgery for ovarian cancer. *British Medical Journal*, **302**, 259–62.

Fox, H. (1985). Pathology of surface epithelial tumours. In *Ovarian cancer* (ed. C. N. Hudson), pp. 72–93. Oxford University Press.

Gadducci, A., Bruzzone, M., Carnio, F. *et al.* (1996). Twelve year follow-up of a randomized trial comparing cisplatin and cyclophosphamide with cisplatin, doxorubicin and cyclophosphamide in patients with advanced epithelial ovarian cancer. *International Journal of Gynecological Cancer*, **6**, 286–90.

Gore, M. E., Fryatt, I., Wiltshaw, E., and Dawson, T. (1990). Treatment of relapsed carcinoma of the ovary with cisplatin or carboplatin following initial treatment with these compounds. *Gynecologic Oncology*, **36**, 207–11.

Hird, V., Maraveyas, A., Snook, D. *et al.* (1993). Adjuvant therapy of ovarian cancer with radioactive monoclonal antiboty. *British Journal of Cancer*, **68**, 403–6.

Jacobs, I. (1995). Screening for sporadic ovarian cancer. In *The biology of gynaecological cancer* (ed. R. Leak, M. Gore, and R. H. Ward), pp. 231–44. RCOG Press, London.

Jacobs, I. J., Skates, S., Prys Davies, A. *et al.* (1996). Risk of diagnosis of ovarian cancer after raised serum CA 125 concentration: a prospective cohort study. *British Medical Journal*, **313**, 1355–8.

Kaern, J., Trope, C. G., Kristensen, V. M. *et al.* (1993). DNA ploidy; the most important prognostic factor in patients with borderline tumors of the ovary. *International Journal of Gynecological Cancer*, **3**, 349–58.

Lambert, H. E. and Berry, R. J. (1985). High dose cisplatin compared with high dose cyclophosphamide in the management of advanced epithelial ovarian cancer Stage III and IV: a report from the North Thames Co-operative Group. *British Medical Journal*, **290**, 889–93.

Lambert, H. E., Rustin, G., Gregory, W., and Nelstrop, A. (1993). A randomised trial comparing single agent carboplatin with carboplatin followed by radiotherapy for advanced ovarian cancer: A North Thames Ovary Group Study. *Journal of Clinical Oncology*, **11**, 440–8.

Marks, J. R., Davidoff, A. M., Kerns, D. J. M. *et al.* (1991). Overexpression and mutation of p53 in epithelial ovarian cancer. *Cancer Research*, **51**, 2979–84.

McGuire, W. P., Hoskins, W. J., Brady, M. F. *et al.* (1996). Cyclophosphamide and cisplatin compared with Paclitaxel and cisplatin in patients with Stage III and Stage IV ovarian cancer. *New England Journal of Medicine*, **334**, 1–6.

Newlands, E. S. and Bagshaw, K. D. (1987). Advances in the treatment of germ cell tumours of the ovary. In *Recent advances in obstetrics and gynaecology* (ed. J. Bonnar), pp. 143–56. Churchill Livingstone, Edinburgh.

Ovarian Cancer Meta-analysis Project (1991). Cyclophosphamide, doxorubicin and cisplatin chemotherapy of ovarian carcinoma: A meta-analysis. *Journal of Clinical Oncology*, **9**, 1668–74.

Ovarian Tumour Panel of the Royal College of Obstetricians and Gynaecologists (1983). Ovarian epithelial tumours of borderline malignancy: pathological features and current status. *British Journal of Obstetrics and Gynaecology*, **90**, 743–50.

Sjovall, K., Nilsson, B., and Einhorn, N. (1994). Different types of rupture of the tumour capsule and the impact on survival in early ovarian carcinoma. *International Journal of Gynecological Cancer*, **4**, 333–6.

Teilum, G. (1965). Classification of endodermal sinus tumours (mesoblastoma vitellinum) and so called 'embyonal carcinoma' of the ovary. *Act Pathologica Microgiologica*, **64**, 407.

Van Dam, P. A., Vergote, I. B., Lowe, D. G. *et al.* (1993). Epidermal growth factor receptor expression is an independent prognostic factor in ovarian cancer. *International Journal of Gynecological Cancer*, **3**(Suppl. 1), 15.

Van der Berg, M. E. L. *et al.* (1995). The effect of debulking surgery after induction chemotherapy on the prognosis in advanced epithelial ovarian cancer. *New England Journal of Medicine*, **332**, 629–34.

Vergote, I. B., De Vos, L. N., Abeler, V. M. *et al.* (1992). Randomised trial comparing cisplatin with radioactive phosphorus or whole abdominal irradiation as adjuvant treatment of ovarian cancer. *Cancer*, **69**, 741–9.

Vergote, I. B., Trope, C. G., Kaern, J. *et al.* (1993). Identification of high-risk stage I ovarian carcinoma. Importance of DNA ploidy. *International Journal of Gynecological Cancer*, **3**(Suppl. 1), 51.

Vessey, M., Metcalf, A., Wells, C. *et al.* (1987). Ovarian neoplasms, functional cysts and oral contraceptives. *British Medical Journal*, **294**, 1518–20.

Watson, P. and Lynch, H. T. (1992). *Hereditary ovarian cancer*, Vol. 2: *Biology, diagnosis and management*, (ed. F. Sharp, W. P. Mason, and W. Creasman), pp. 9–15. Chapman and Hall, London.

Yates, J. R. W. (1996). Medical genetics. *British Medical Journal*, **312**, 1021–5.

Young, R. C., Chabner, B. A., Hubbard, S. P. *et al.* (1978). Advanced ovarian adenocarcinoma: a prospective clinical trial of melphelan (L-PAM) versus combination chemotherapy. *New England Journal of Medicine*, **299**, 1261–6.

Young, R. C., Walton, L. A., Ellenberg, S. S. *et al.* (1990). Adjuvant therapy in stage I and stage II epithelial ovarian cancer: results of two prospective randomized trials. *New England Journal of Medicine*, **322**, 1021–7.

3

Cancer of the cervix

Incidence and epidemiology

In England and Wales there are almost 4500 new cases of cancer of the cervix per annum. The incidence of invasive cancer of the cervix in the UK appears to be falling but there has been a marked increase in the number of women diagnosed with pre-invasive cancer (cervical intra-epithelial neoplasia, CIN III) which now outnumbers invasive cervical cancer by a factor of nearly 5:1. The peak incidence of pre-invasive lesions occurs between the ages of 25 and 40 years. Although the incidence of cervical cancer has risen in women aged 25–34, the peak incidence is in the 45–50 year age group.

World-wide cervical cancer is the second most common female malignancy after breast cancer and its incidence far exceeds that of either cancer of the ovary or endometrium. This incidence varies between countries. It is the commonest female cancer in many developing areas and in India cervical cancer is the commonest cause of death in women aged 35–45 years. In the UK the lifetime risk of developing cancer of the cervix is 1.3 percent, while in Columbia it is 5.5 percent, but only 0.5 percent in Spain and Israel.

There are also epidemiological differences between different socio-economic groups within a country. In the USA, black women have almost twice the risk of developing cancer of the cervix as white women. This difference is not thought to be because of ethnic group, but due to the fact that black women are more likely to be in the lower socio-economic groups. A study in the west of Scotland showed a similar result, with women from low income families having a threefold increased risk of developing cervical cancer compared to more affluent groups (Lammont *et al.* 1993).

There is a falling rate in the incidence rate of invasive cervical cancer in North America and Scandinavia, as well as in the UK, and this is associated with a reduced mortality. While this lower rate of invasive cervical cancer can be attributed to the detection of pre-invasive lesions through widespread screening, some of the fall in the incidence of cancer of the cervix preceded the establishment of screening programmes.

Aetiology

Although there is increasing evidence for a viral aetiology for the development of cervical cancer, there are probably several risk factors which are also involved. Some of the risk factors which have been found to be associated with cancer of the cervix, include sexual behaviour, parity, smoking, and genital wart disease.

Sexual behaviour

While cancer of the cervix can occur in any woman, two aspects of sexual behaviour: early age at first intercourse and a high number of sexual partners of the female, appear to be risk factors (Brinton *et al.* 1987). There is a higher incidence of both pre-invasive cervical intra-epithelial neoplasia and of invasive disease in women who commenced regular intercourse in their teens compared to those who did not commence until a later age. This suggests that the adolescent cervix may be more vulnerable to transmissable oncogenic agents.

The relative risk of a woman developing cervical neoplasia also seems to be increased if the male partner has had multiple sexual partners, although this association has not been verified by a Swedish study (Hellberg and Nilsson 1989).

Contraception

The effect of contraception on the risk of developing cancer of the cervix appears to be minimal. It has been suggested that oral contraceptives increase the risk but the increased rate of cervical intra-epithelial neplasia (CIN) found in women taking oral contraceptives may be related to improved detection rates, as a result of more regular screening (Irwin *et al.* 1988).

Smoking

An association has been shown between smoking and cervical neoplasia. Smoking may increase the risk of developing cervical neoplasia both directly and indirectly (Barton *et al.* 1988). The evidence for a direct effect is that the products of smoking have been found to be concentrated in the cervical mucus and smoking can produce changes in the DNA of cervical squamous cells. The indirect effect is that smoking can cause a degree of immuno-suppression by decreasing the population of Langerhan's cells responsible for cell-mediated immunity in the cervix, thus rendering the cervix more vulnerable to infection by a transmissable agent.

Immunosuppression

Systemic immunosuppression appears to increase the risk of CIN. For example, CIN is more common in women who have undergone renal trans-plant, or who are HIV positive. Invasive squamous cell carcinoma of the cervix, in an HIV positive woman, is an AIDS indicator disease.

Viral infections

Viral infections appear to play an important role in the genesis of cervical neoplasia. Human papilloma viruses (HPV), have attracted most attention in recent years. Over 70 types of HPV have been isolated of which over 20 are associated with the lower genital tract. HPV 16, 18, 31, and 33 are the main oncological viruses (see Chapter 7, p. 144 on molecular biology).

HPV 16 appears to be present in 90–100 percent of invasive squamous cell cancers and HPV 18 is associated with adenocarcinoma of the cervix. In an epidemiological study in Finland of nearly 19 000 women followed for 23 years, women with serological evidence of having been infected with HPV 16, showed an excess risk of cervical cancer (Lehtinen *et al.* 1996). As not all women with the human papilloma virus (HPV 16) develop cervical neoplasia, it has been postulated that normal women may eradicate the virus without developing neoplasia, whereas the women in whom the virus persists are at risk (Munoz *et al.* 1988). Tests are being carried out on a vaccine against HPV 16 and 18 which could result in a significant fall in the incidence of cervical cancer in the future.

Herpes simplex virus 2 (HSV 2) was once considered to be the infective agent for cervical cancer. This view is no longer held, although it may have a role as a co-factor.

Anatomy

The uterus is a muscular organ comprising a body (the corpus) and a neck (the cervix). The cervix projects into the vagina. The endocervical canal connects the cavity of the uterus with the vagina (Fig. 3.1). The size of the body of the uterus and the cervix alter with age, being small before puberty,

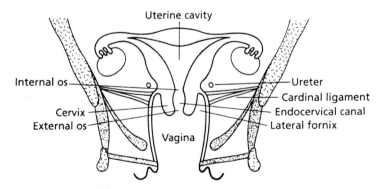

Fig. 3.1 Anatomical relationships of the cervix including the ureters and cardinal ligaments (parametria).

growing to approximately 7 cm long overall during childbearing years, and then shrinking after the menopause.

The uterovesical ligaments lie anteriorly but do not contribute significantly to uterine support. The cervix lies above and in continuity with the vagina and is posterior to the bladder and anterior to the rectum and pouch of Douglas (Fig. 3.2). Cranially, it is in continuity with the body of the uterus, and is also related to the peritoneum and the contents of the pelvis. The cervix is supported by the cardinal ligaments laterally and uterosacral ligaments posteriorly (Fig. 3.3). Laterally the cervix abuts the paracervical tissues, the broad ligaments, and the ureters which run close to its lateral margins.

The function of the cervix is to act as a sphincter. It is involved in conception and then maintains the integrity of the uterine cavity during pregnancy. In labour the sphincter action is reversed to allow delivery of the fetus.

Squamocolumnar junction

The squamocolumnar junction is the junction between the squamous epithelium covering the ectocervix and the columnar epithelium lining the cervical canal. It is situated just inside the external cervical os in young women, rising up the endocervical canal after the menopause. At adolescence and first pregnancy, with hormone stimulation, the cervix grows and everts exposing the thin glandular epithelium of the endocervical canal. This

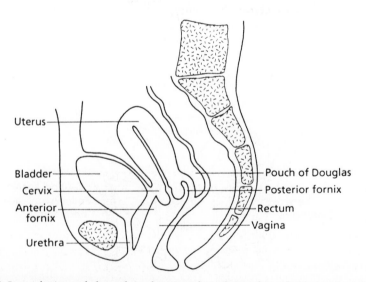

Fig. 3.2 Lateral view of the pelvis showing the relationship of the cervix to the bladder, rectum, and pouch of Douglas.

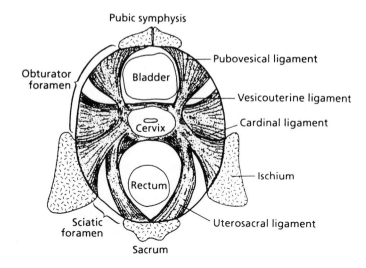

Fig. 3.3 The supporting ligaments of the uterus at the level of the cervix.

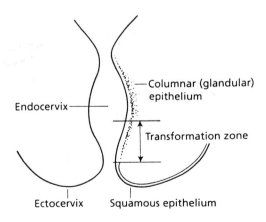

Fig. 3.4 Transformation zone of the cervix.

exposed epithelium is gradually replaced by squamous epithelium by a process known as *squamous metaplasia* and the part of the cervix which is lined by this metaplastic squamous epithelium is known as the *transformation zone* (Fig. 3.4).

Cervical squamous neoplasia arise in the transformation zone. The increased risk of developing cervical neoplasia, associated with regular sexual intercourse in the teenage years, may be due to the transformation zone being exposed at an early age to transmissable agents such as oncogenic viruses.

Lymphatic drainage

The regional lymph drainage of the female genital organs follows a relatively well-defined pattern. Direct drainage occurs to the parametrial glands and to the obturator, internal, external, and common iliac nodes. Drainage to the pre-sacral nodes can also occur (Fig. 3.5). Spread to the para-aortic nodes is rare without pelvic node involvement. The supraclavicular nodes may be involved in advanced disease.

Spread of disease

Carcinoma of the cervix spreads predominantly by direct invasion and by lymphatic permeation. Direct spread is to the vaginal mucosa inferiorly, and via the endocervical canal to the uterine cavity superiorly. Laterally, the parametrial tissues and ligaments of the uterus may be involved and this involvement can extend to the pelvic side wall. The ureters may be invaded or constricted by tumour. In advanced disease, direct spread can involve the bladder anteriorly or the rectum posteriorly. Spread is usually continuous, but seedlings from cervical cancer can occasionally be noted in the lower vagina.

The risk of pelvic lymph node metastases is increased in the presence of lymphatic vessel invasion within the tumour, poor differentiation and large tumour volume. Metastatic blood spread to lungs, bone, and liver is unusual and late and usually only occurs in the presence of locally advanced disease.

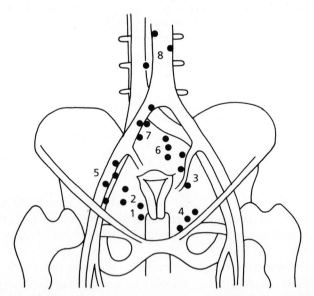

Fig. 3.5 Lymph node drainage of the cervix: (1) paracervical; (2) parametrial; (3) internal iliac; (4) obturator; (5) external iliac; (6) pre-sacral; (7) common iliac; (8) para-aortic.

Pathology

The majority of cervical cancers, 85–95 percent, are squamous cell in origin. Adenocarcinomas, which appear to be increasing in frequency, account for most of the rest.

SQUAMOUS CARCINOMA OF THE CERVIX

Pre-invasive disease (CIN)

Squamous cell carcinoma of the cervix and its precursors arise in the transformation zone where the ectocervical squamous epithelium meets the glandular epithelium of the endocervical canal. If the metaplastic process in the transformation zone is disrupted, dysplastic changes may develop in the epithelium. The terms *CIN I*, *CIN II*, and *CIN III*, are *histological* terms used to describe increasing degrees of dysplasia from mild to severe. Severe dysplasia (CIN III) includes what was previously known as carcinoma *in situ*. The terms broadly correlate with mild, moderate, and severe dyskariosis seen on cervical cytology.

The Bethesda System is used in the USA where CIN II–III lesions are considered as high grade squamous intra-epithelial lesions (HGSIL) and CIN I and HPV changes are considered as low grade squamous intra-epithelial lesions (LGSIL).

As most cases of CIN III lesions are treated, it is difficult to predict how many will become invasive if treatment is not given. A significant minority, about one-third, of cases of CIN I would revert to normal if left untreated but it is considered that up to two-thirds of cases of CIN III has the potential to develop into invasive cancer. At present it is felt acceptable to be conservative in cases of CIN I although careful follow-up is required to detect changes to a high grade lesion. The natural history of CIN is that the development of cancer is usually a slow process which may take 10 to 20 years.

Superficial carcinoma (previously known as *microinvasion*)

As the earlier name implies, the invasion through the basement membrane of the epithelium is only visible microscopically. Tiny prongs of squamous carcinoma are seen infiltrating into the cervical stroma. This microinvasion can occur from either surface epithelium or from involved crypts. This is the earliest stage in the International Federation of Gynaecology and Obstetrics (FIGO) classification for carcinoma of the cervix (*stage Ia*). Stage Ia which includes lesions up to 5 mm in depth and 7 mm in width, is subdivided into state *Ia*1 (up to 3 mm depth) and *Ia*2 (up to 5 mm depth) (Table 3.1). This

Table 3.1 FIGO staging for carcinoma of the cervix

Stage	Features
0	Pre-invasive carcinoma (CIN)
I	**Invasive: confined to the cervix[a]**
Ia	Invasive cancer identified only microscopically.[b] Invasion is limited to measured stromal invasion with a maximum depth of 5 mm[c] and no wider than 7 mm
Ia1	Measured invasion of stroma no greater than 3 mm in depth and no wider than 7 mm diameter
Ia2	Measured invasion of stroma greater than 3 mm and no greater than 5 mm in depth and no wider than 7 mm in diameter
Ib	Clinical lesions confined to the cervix or pre-clinical lesions greater than stage Ia
Ib1	Clinical lesions no greater than 4 cm in size
Ib2	Clinical lesions greater than 4 cm in size
II	**Extenson of cancer beyond cervix into vagina or parametria but not into lower third of vagina or reaching pelvic side wall**
IIa	Carcinoma extending beyond the cervix into the upper two-thirds of the vagina
IIb	Carcinoma extending into the parametria but not reaching the pelvic side wall
III	**Extension of cancer to pelvic side wall or to lower third of vagina**
IIIa	Carcinoma involving the lower third of the vagina but not reaching the pelvic side wall
IIIb	Carcinoma extending to the pelvic side-wall or hydronephrosis or non-functioning kidney[d]
IV	**Extension beyond true pelvis or clinical involvement of mucosa of the bladder and/or rectum**
IVa	Carcinoma involving adjacent organs
IVb	Distant metastasis

FIGO, International Federation of Gynaecology and Obstetrics.
[a] Extension to the uterine corpus is disregarded.
[b] All gross lesions even with superficial invasion are stage Ib.
[c] The depth of invasion should not be more than 5 mm taken from the base of the epithelium, either surface or glandular, from which it originates. Vascular space involvement, either venous or lymphatic, should not alter the staging.
[d] All cases with hydronephrosis or non-functioning kidney are included unless known to be due to other causes.

subdivision reflects the *conservative* surgery required for stage *Ia*1, when nodal involvement is most unlikely.

When the depth of invasion is greater than 5 mm, or the width more than 7 mm, the tumour is *stage Ib*, even if the tumour can only be detected microscopically.

Invasive carcinoma

Most squamous carcinomas involve the ectocervix and are often visible on speculum examination. The tumour may be exophytic or endophytic, and may infiltrate other structures. Ulceration occurs frequently, particularly with the larger tumours.

Squamous cell carcinomas of the cervix are usually classified according to their degree of differentiation: well-differentiated (grade 1/G1); moderately differentiated (grade 2/G2); and poorly differentiated (grade 3/G3). Alternative classification of squamous cell tumours is that of the World Health Organization (WHO), which subdivides tumours into three groups namely, keratinizing, large-cell non-keratinizing, and small cell non-keratinizing.

Screening

Pre-invasive disease, cervical intra-epithelial neoplasia, is asymptomatic but cytological examination of a cervical smear can show abnormalities. The cervix can then be examined by low amplification microscopy using a colposcope and any abnormal areas detected can be biopsied for histological assessment.

The ease and reliability of cervical cytology has resulted in screening programmes in several countries. In communities such as British Columbia, Iceland, and Finland regular, widespread screening in the 1960s and 1970s resulted in a marked reduction in the overall incidence and mortality of cervical cancer by detecting the disease in the pre-invasive stage of the disease (Table 3.2). In other countries, such as the UK, a less marked decrease in mortality was seen due to a poorer compliance rate (Sirgurdsson, 1993). Improvements in the organization of the service occurred in the UK in 1988 with the setting up of an NHS cervical screening programme co-ordinating network and the introduction of a systematic call–recall system. Screening is recommended for women aged 20–60 years and 83 percent of the target population were screened between 1992 and 1994 (Austoker 1994). There will always be difficulties in providing screening for the whole target population, especially as women at highest risk do not always avail themselves of the service. However, the effect of more widespread screening is now leading to a significant reduction in mortality in the UK from cancer of the cervix. In developing countries the cost of mass screening is too great for it to be carried out on a national scale.

Table 3.2 Effectiveness of screening for cancer of the cervix (1960s–1970s)

	Finland	Iceland
Target cover of national population	100%	100%
Target age	30–55 years	25–69 years
Screening interval	5 years	2–3 years
Reduction in overall world adjusted incidence rate	66%	70%
Reduction in overall world mortality rate	60%	62%

Procedure for taking a cervical smear

A cervical smear is performed as follows: a sample of cells is obtained from the ectocervix, transformation zone, and endocervix by scraping the surface with a wooden or plastic spatula. The most commonly used are wooden (the Ayre's or Aylesbury spatula with an extended tip) or plastic (Rocket) spatulas. The pointed part of the spatula is inserted into the cervical canal and then the spatula is rotated through 720 degrees (Fig. 3.6). The smear obtained is spread on to a microscope slide and immediately fixed with alcohol to prevent air-drying. The cells are stained by the Papanicolau technique and then examined in the laboratory. For a satisfactory smear, squamous cells and at least two of the following: metaplastic cells, endo-cervical cells, or endocervical mucus must be present.

Terminology for cervical cytology

The terminology used for cervical cytology and its interpretation is shown on Table 3.3. There is a continuous range of cytological abnormalities from normal to malignant. The abnormal appearances in the cells are described as dyskaryosis, mild, moderate, and severe. The relationship between cytology and histology is also shown on Table 3.3. As the smear is only a sample of cells from the transformation zone, the underlying histology is the more significant.

HPV typing

At present in the UK, cervical cytology alone is offered for screening although the use of HPV typing may be helpful in more accurately

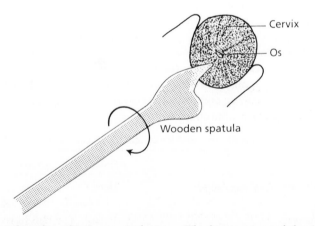

Fig. 3.6 Procedure for taking a cervical smear. The long tongue of the Aylesbury spatula is pushed well into the cervical os before rotating the spatula through 720 degrees to obtain cells from the transformation zone for cytological examination.

Table 3.3 Cytology reports and relationship to histological findings and suggested action

Cytology	Histology		Action
Normal[a]	CIN II/III	<1%	Repeat 3-yearly
Inflammatory changes	CIN II/III	10%	*No consensus*
			Repeat smear in 6 months.
			Colposcopy if lesion persists
Borderline nuclear changes + or − HPV changes	CIN II/III	20–40%	Repeat smear in 6 months. Colposcopy if lesion persists[b]
Mild dyskariosis + or − HPV changes	CIN II/III	50%	As above[b]
Moderate dyskariosis + or − HPV changes	CIN II/III	50–70%	Colposcopy
Severe dyskariosis + or − HPV changes	CIN II/III	80–90%	Colposcopy
	Invasive	5%	
Invasion	Invasive	50%	Urgent investigation
Abnormal glandular cells	Possible adenocarcinoma *in in situ*/adenocarcinomas of the cervix or endometrium		Urgent investigation

[a] Smears reported as inadequate must always be repeated.
[b] A minimum of 2 consecutive negative smears at least 6 months apart are required before returning to 3-yearly screening.
Table modified from Soutter (1993).

predicting histology from the cytology of the cervical smear. In a study by Cuzik *et al.* (1992) almost all of the 85 women presenting with low grade cytological abnormalities and who also had a significant amount of HPV 16, were subsequently found to have high grade CIN.

Frequency of cervical screening

The frequency of cervical screening needed to ensure maximum detection rates of pre-invasive cervical cancer, is a matter of debate. In the UK, the present recommendation is to screen women aged 20–60 years every 3 to 5 years.

Colposcopy

Colposcopy involves examining the cervix with low-power binocular microscopy. By staining the cervix and upper vagina with acetic acid and then iodine, areas of abnormal epithelium which are stained differentially are identified. An alternative staining method using saline can be used to detect abnormal vasculature. These methods allow precise definition of those areas that need to be biopsied.

Cervicography

After applying acetic acid to the cervix, a colposcopic photograph is taken. The results can be screened at high speed by trained personnel who decide which women need further investigation. Cervicography has been shown to be more accurate, but also more expensive, than cytology. Its use is not widespread at present.

Clinical features of invasive cancer of the cervix

Symptoms and signs

The most common symptom of invasive cervical cancer is abnormal vaginal bleeding. This can be postcoital, intermenstrual, or postmenopausal. The second commonest symptom is an offensive vaginal discharge. Pain, described as a dragging sensation, in the pelvis or referred leg pain only occurs in advanced cases with nerve and muscle involvement. In locally advanced disease (stage IVa), spread into the bladder may cause frequency of micturition and haematuria. Spread of tumour into the rectum is rare, but if present, can cause tenesmus and rectal bleeding. Very early cervical cancer, detected by screening, may be asymptomatic.

The cervix may be enlarged, have obvious growth on its surface or be ulcerated. Tumour may extend to the vagina or, more rarely, to the vulva. Involvement of the parametria may be detected. Nodal masses may be present on the pelvic side walls or in more advanced cases, in the abdomen, inguinal regions or left supraclavicular fossa. Rarely, signs of a deep vein thrombosis of the lower limbs or lymphoedema are present.

Clinical examination

Examination of the patient should include palpation of the abdomen for hydronephrosis and hepatomegaly, and for nodal involvement (para-aortic, inguinal, and supraclavicular). The vulva, vagina, and cervix should be inspected. If a suspicious lesion is seen, cytology and a biopsy should be taken.

Bimanual examination, that is with one hand on the abdomen and two fingers in the vagina allows assessment of the size, shape, and mobility of the uterus and palpation of the adnexae and of any extension of tumour into the surrounding tissues. Rectal examination is essential to assess posterior spread of the tumour along the uterosacral ligaments, parametrial invasion, and involvement of nodes on the pelvic side wall. Under anaesthetic, the parametria may be better examined with the index finger in the vagina and the middle finger in the rectum.

Investigations

Examination under anaesthesia

Examination under anaesthesia (EUA) is an essential investigation for all cases of carcinoma of the cervix, even when the diagnosis is known. This is to allow the extent of the disease to be accurately staged and to enable the treatment to be defined.

Ideally, EUA should be performed jointly by the gynaecologist and clinical oncologist treating the patient. Abdominal examination followed by pelvic examination are carried out as detailed above, and, in addition, cystoscopy is necessary to rule out bladder involvement. Bullous oedema of the bladder mucosa may be present with advanced cervical cancer but, unless tumour is seen, this is not sufficient to make the patient stage IVa (Table 3.1). If there is any suspicion of rectal spread, proctoscopy and sigmoidoscopy should be part of the procedure.

The cervix is biopsied if a histological diagnosis of cancer of cervix has not already been made. Any further abnormal areas in the vagina or vulva are biopsied. Usually a sample of endometrium is obtained although endometrial involvement does not change the management of the patient.

Radiological tests

Radiological imaging of the renal tract is a requirement for FIGO staging as evidence of ureteric obstruction or stenosis is one of the defining features of stage IIIb. An intravenous urogram (IVU) is the minimum investigation required, but in the UK a CT scan is more commonly performed. This scan will also assess the liver, para-aortic and pelvic lymph nodes and direct spread within the pelvis. Magnetic resonance imaging (MRI) is a valuable tool for assessing spread in the parametrium and nodal involvement. However, no radiological technique, even lymphography, is particularly accurate at assessing pelvic node involvement. Fine needle aspiration of suspicious nodes may confirm the presence of positive nodes but in early stage disease, histological examination of the nodes removed at pelvic lymphadenectomy, is the only accurate way of determining nodal involvement.

Tumour markers

Tumour markers such as CA125, CA19-9, carcino-embryonic antigen (CEA), and the squamous cell carcinoma antigen (SCC), which have been shown to be raised in cervical cancer, correlate with stage, volume of disease and the presence of nodal metastases. They are not, at present, routinely used in clinical practice.

Clinical staging

FIGO (International Federation of Gynaecology and Obstetrics) staging is the standard system used world-wide for gynaecological tumours. The FIGO staging for cancer of the cervix is shown in Table 3.1. Except for Stage Ia, which is defined histologically, the staging is *clinical* based on the findings at EUA. Urological and chest radiography are also used when determining the FIGO stage, but abnormal nodal findings or possible parametrial involvement from other imaging techniques do not affect the FIGO staging.

Prognostic factors

More than 90 percent of patients with stage I tumours, with uninvolved lymph nodes, can be cured but results remain disappointing for advanced tumours, with 5-year survival rates of only 30 percent for stage III and less than 10 percent for stage IV (Table 3.4). The main prognostic findings include tumour volume, stage and nodal involvement, all of which are inter-related.

Stage and volume

Stage is the single most important prognostic factor. Tumour volume is of major significance and this factor has led to recent changes in the FIGO system. Stage Ib is now divided into: stage Ib1, tumours smaller or equal to 4 cm in diameter; and stage Ib2, tumours more than 4 cm in diameter. The wide range in tumour size in stage Ib from microscopic disease greater than that in stage Ia to diameters of up to 8 cm is shown in Fig. 3.7.

The FIGO system of staging takes no account of endometrial involvement in stage I disease, despite the fact that an increased tumour volume is associated with a poorer prognosis. Similarly, in both stage IIb and IIIb, no differentiation exists between unilateral and bilateral spread despite the poorer prognosis with the latter. Figure 3.8 demonstrates the findings in stage IIa to IVa cancer of the cervix.

The incidence of pelvic and para-aortic nodal metastases rises with

Table 3.4 Results of treatment of cervical carcinoma (modified from FIGO 1988)

Stage	% of total	5-year survival (%)
I	35	76
II	34	55
III	26	30
IV	4	7

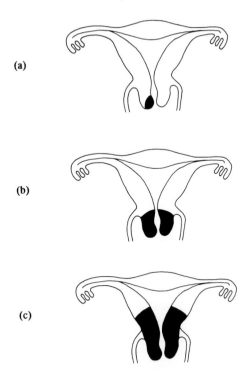

(a)

(b)

(c)

Fig. 3.7 Stage Ib tumour carcinoma of the cervix demonstrating how this stage includes a wide range of volumes from (a) Ib1 minimal disease to (b) bulky Ib1 tumours <4 cm; and (c) Ib2 tumour involving the whole cervix and extending into the uterine body.

increasing tumour stage (Table 3.5). Nodal status has a profound effect on survival. In patients with Stage Ib tumours with positive nodes, the 5-year survival is approximately 45 percent, half that of patients with negative nodes. Involvement of para-aortic nodes is usually a marker of widespread dissemination and very few patients are alive 5 years after diagnosis.

Lymphovascular involvement

Lymphovascular space involvement is of prognostic significance in that it is an indicator of probable lymph node involvement.

Histology

Although some series suggest that poorly differentiated squamous cell carcinomas have a worse prognosis than more differentiated tumours, other studies have been unable to find histological grade to be significant. Cervical adenocarcinomas are considered to have a worse prognosis than squamous

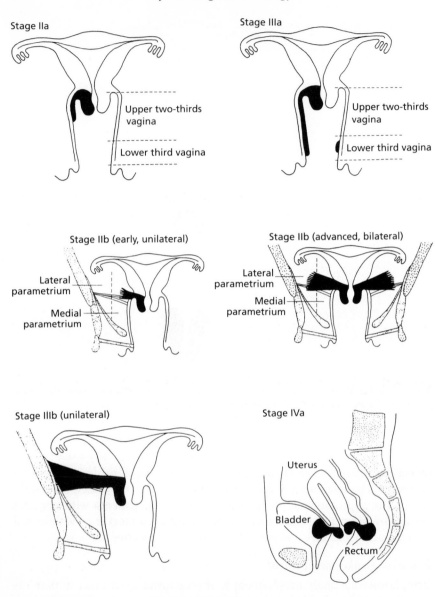

Fig. 3.8 Stages II–IVa carcinoma of the cervix.

carcinomas, but they arise in the endocervical canal and are usually advanced at diagnosis. The very rare small cell neuroendocrine and oat cell tumours of the cervix have a particularly bad prognosis because early lymphatic and haematogenous spread commonly occurs.

Table 3.5 Incidence of nodal involvement

Stage	Positive pelvic nodes (%)	Positive para-aortic nodes (%)
Ib	16	7
II	30	16
III	44	35
IV	55	40

HPV status

HPV viruses can suppress the action of the normal (wild) type of the tumour suppressor gene *p53*. Patients with HPV positive squamous carcinoma of the cervix, however, have a better prognosis than patients who have HPV negative tumours expressing mutant *p53*.

Age

The peak age for developing cancer of the cervix is 45–50 years, but it can occur in women in the third decade of life. While some reports have shown no effect of age on prognosis others have found that young age carries a worse prognosis.

Treatment of CIN and superficial squamous carcinoma (stage Ia)

Cervical intra-epithelial neoplasia (CIN) I–III

CIN I may be managed conservatively if adequate follow-up can be assured. CIN II–III is usually treated by excision under colposcopic control.

The area treated should include the whole of the 'active' transformation zone, that is, the central part of the ectocervix which is covered by metaplastic epithelium or CIN, with a 2 mm margin. In order to include the cervical glands, which may also be affected, treatment should ideally extend to at least 7 mm and preferably 10 mm below the surface.

Treatment for CIN is preferably by excision but ablative techniques are also used. Excision has the advantage over ablation in that it allows histological confirmation of complete excision of the area of CIN and that an invasive lesion has not been missed. Excisional therapy can be by electrodiathermy loop (LLETZ), laser surgery, or scalpel. Cone biopsy of the cervix is carried out where lesions extend into the endocervical canal, the extent of which is not visible on colposcopic examination, to ensure their complete removal, and for superficial carcinoma. Ablation is carried out under colposcopic control by radical electrodiathermy, cold coagulation, cryotherapy or carbon dioxide laser vaporization (see Chapter 8, p. 157).

Results of treatment of the cervix for CIN are very good with reported cure rates of 90–95 percent regardless of the modality used.

Follow-up

At present, the UK guidelines suggest a follow up colposcopy and smear at 6 months post-treatment. If normal, cervical cytology is then performed at 1 year post-treatment and thereafter annually. If the cytology is negative for 3 years, the woman may return to the normal screening programme.

Superficial carcinoma of the cervix: FIGO stage Ia

A cone biopsy is required to make the initial diagnosis of superficial invasion. Cone biopsy which completely excises a stage *Ia1* lesion is sufficient treatment as the danger of lymph node metastases is less than 0.5 percent. It is inappropriate to perform hysterectomy as treatment until the definitive diagnosis is made.

For the lesions included in stage *Ia2* where the depth of invasion is 3–5 mm, the possibility of node involvement is approximately 7 percent. The presence of lymphatic space involvement and confluence is also considered to increase the likelihood of lymph node involvement being present.

In the UK, it would be considered acceptable to treat a stage Ia2 lesion with a cone biopsy, which completely removes the lesion, in those women who wished to preserve their fertility. In the USA and Japan, radical hysterectomy and pelvic lymphadenectomy would be the treatment of choice. However, this may be overtreatment.

Treatment of invasive cervical cancer

The definitive treatment for invasive cancer of the cervix is either surgery or radiotherapy. The survival rate is equivalent for both modalities. The choice of treatment will depend on the stage, size, and histology of the tumour, the risk of lymph node involvement and the fitness of the patient. In some cases both forms of treatment are used and chemotherapy may be added. The treatment regimen should be decided after joint consultation between the gynaecological and clinical oncologist.

Surgery

Surgery is the treatment of choice in women who have stage Ib cancer of the cervix, in whom the risk of nodal metastases is low. Nodal involvement is unlikely if the tumour is of small volume (<4 cm), well or moderately differentiated with no lymphatic vessel invasion, and there is no imaging evidence of enlarged nodes.

The surgical procedure is a *radical hysterectomy and pelvic lymph-*

adenctomy (see Chapter 8, p. 160). In a radical hysterectomy, the uterus, upper vagina, and parametria are excised together with the pelvic lymph nodes. The ovaries can be conserved in premenopausal women thus avoiding an early menopause. Age and obesity are not contraindications to radical surgery.

The advantages for women having radical surgery rather than radio-therapy are the retention of a pliable and lubricated vagina, the absence of menopausal symptoms in premenopausal women, and the avoidance of the small risk of a late radiation-induced second malignancy. In addition, accurate surgical staging of disease gives clear prognostic information that can influence further management. Generally, surgery is used for stage Ib1 and radiotherapy for stage Ib2 although in individual cases surgery may be appropriate for both stage Ib2 and IIa.

Radiotherapy

Radiotherapy is the treatment of choice for women with stage Ib cancer of the cervix who are not suitable for radical surgery or when the surgical expertise to perform radical hysterectomy is not available. Radiotherapy is also used as primary treatment in women at high risk of nodal involvement. The factors associated with nodal involvement have already been listed and include large volume tumours, poor tumour differentiation, and lymphatic vessel involvement. Such patients are unlikely to be cured by surgery as complete excision is often not possible due to metastatic spread. Unfortunately, even small doses of radiotherapy will ablate the ovarian function and hormone replacement therapy is then necessary.

Carcinoma of the cervix is treated by a course of external radiotherapy to the whole pelvis, followed by intracavitary brachytherapy where radio-therapy sources are placed into the uterine cavity and upper vagina. In non-bulky, early stage cancer of the cervix, treatment in some cancer centres is by intracavitary therapy alone. A maximum diameter of 3 centimetres would usually be regarded as the limit of size for a tumour to be treated by intracavitary brachytherapy only.

External beam therapy

The volume treated by external radiation will include the tumour and the pelvic nodes which drain the cervix, that is, the external, internal, and common iliac nodes (see Figure 3.5). The pelvic volume can be encompassed by treating with 2 fields, anteriorly and posteriorly, or with 3 fields—one anterior and two lateral or posterior-lateral in order to spare the posterior wall of the rectum, or in obese patients with 4 fields, anterior, posterior, and two lateral.

The anterior and posterior treatment fields will extend superiorly from

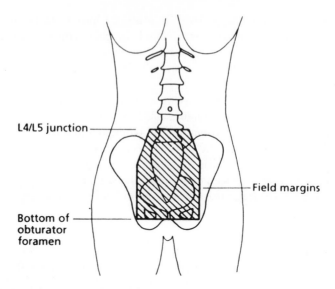

L4/L5 junction

Field margins

Bottom of
obturator
foramen

Fig. 3.9 The anterior external beam radiotherapy field used to treat carcinoma of
the cervix. The field extends from the junction of the 4th and 5th lumbar vertebrae
to the bottom of the obturator foramina.

the junction of the fourth and fifth lumbar vertebra, to include the upper
common iliac nodes or, alternatively, from the junction of the fifth lumbar
vertebra with the sacrum, and inferiorly to the bottom of the obturator
foramina. Laterally, these treatment fields extend to 1 cm outside the bony
margin of the pelvis (Fig. 3.9). If the position of the lymph nodes is known
from imaging, the upper corners of the volume can be shielded to protect
small bowel. If the tumour involves the vagina the inferior margin is
extended to cover the whole of the involved mucosa with a 2 cm margin.
When lateral fields are used the treatment volume usually extends from the
pubic symphysis anteriorly to the front of S2/S3 junction posteriorly.

Megavoltage, using a 5–8 MeV (mega electron volt) linear accelerator, is
required to deliver radiation at depth, in order to ensure an even distribution of dose within the tumour volume with maximum sparing of the
bladder, rectum, and other normal tissues outside the treatment volume
(Fig. 3.10).

Occasionally, the pelvic field is extended to include the para-aortic nodes,
if these are known to be involved in patients with early disease (stages I–IIa).
The use of multi-leaf collimators allows treatment fields to be tailored to
reduce the risk of radiation damage to the small bowel and kidneys. There is
no evidence that treating the para-aortic nodes, in the presence of *locally
advanced* disease (stages IIb–IV), improves survival.

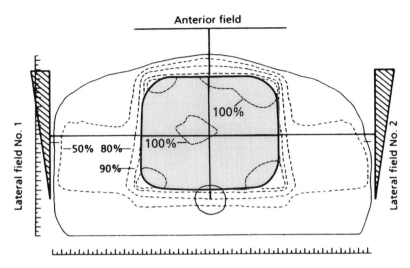

Fig. 3.10 The final plan, using an anterior and two wedged lateral fields, to deliver a homogenous dose to the tumour volume to include the primary tumour and the draining lymph nodes.

Intracavitary brachytherapy

Carcinoma of the cervix was one of the first tumours to be treated by radiotherapy. Several systems for intracavitary brachytherapy were developed in the 1920s and 1930s, most notably in Paris, Stockholm, and Manchester, to deliver consistent treatment. This allowed the effectiveness and morbidity of treatment to be measured (see Chapter 9, p. 185).

The Manchester system is the most widely used in the UK. This method, using various sizes of uterine tube and two vaginal ovoids, has been designed to give a constant dose rate of 0.54 Gy per hour to a geometric point 'A' (Figure 9.4, p. 179), by varying the proportion and distribution of the radioactive isotope within each source. (See Chapter 9, p. 176 on units of measurement.) The arrangement of an intrauterine tube with the two ovoids placed in the vaginal fornices (Fig. 3.11a, b) gives a flattened 'pear-shaped' distribution of isodose curves (Fig. 9.13, p. 192). This delivers a very high dose of radiation to the cervix and immediate surrounding tissue as well as increasing the dose to the lymph nodes beyond the cervix whilst, at the same time, reducing the dose received by the rectum and bladder. This arrangement is preferable to the isodose distribution from a single central source extending into the vagina.

Intracavitary brachytherapy can be delivered at various dose rates depending on the activity of the sources used. The dose rates are classified into low, medium, and high (Table 3.6) and, almost universally, the systems

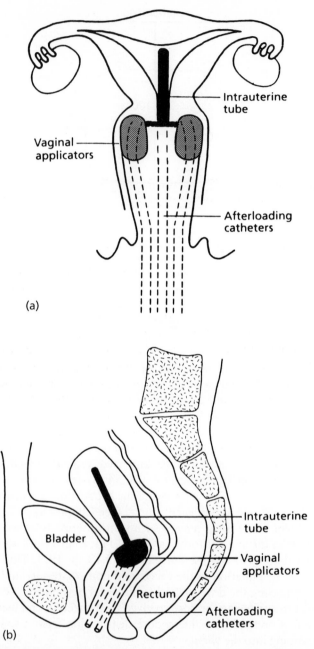

Fig. 3.11 Arrangement of brachytherapy sources for the treatment of carcinoma of the cervix (a) anterior-posterior view of intrauterine tube and vaginal applicators (b) lateral view.

Table 3.6 Definition of intracavitary dose
rate to prescription point (ICRU 1984)

Dose rate	Gray
Low	0.4–2 Gy/hour
Medium	2–12 Gy/hour
High	>0.2 Gy/minute

ICRU, International Commission On Radiological Units.

used fall into the low and high dose rate definitions. This is discussed in detail in Chapter 9 on radiotherapy.

Integration of external beam therapy and intracavitary brachytherapy

The usual radiotherapy treatment for cancer of the cervix is a course of external radiotherapy to the pelvis with additional intracavitary brachytherapy to the cervix and upper vagina. Brachytherapy, which can be given before or after external radiation, allows a higher dose of radiation to be given to the cervix and upper vagina than would be tolerated by the whole pelvis. Classically, intracavitary brachytherapy was given prior to external radiotherapy in order to reduce the tumour mass, with the external beam therapy topping up the dose to the pelvic side walls. With this technique central shielding is needed, in the external beam anterior and posterior fields, to protect the normal tissues (bladder and the rectum) that have already received a high brachytherapy dose. The shielding blocks can be rectangular, a shape which is suitable to shield tissues irradiated by a linear source arrangement. However, this matches the pear-shaped isodose patterns of radiation created by the Manchester system poorly (Fig. 9.13, p. 192). Individual shielding to match these pear-shaped isodoses can be carried out with custom-made blocks or multi-leaf collimators but the exact placement of these shields is difficult and under- or overdosage of one side of the pelvis can occur. This method of treatment is used in some centres for treating early carcinoma of the cervix but is no longer used for advanced disease.

Typically, external beam therapy is used *prior* to intracavitary brachytherapy. This allows a uniform dose of radiation to be received by the pelvis from external radiotherapy and avoids the need for central shielding. This technique is essential in advanced disease to ensure an adequate dose has been received by both the parametria and the pelvic nodes. It also produces shrinkage of the tumour so that subsequent brachytherapy should completely encompass any residual tumour.

Radiotherapy combined with surgery

In the UK the aim of primary treatment is to use only one radical treatment modality but rarely, in bulky disease, following external radiotherapy to the pelvis to reduce the size of the tumour, this is followed by surgery to remove central disease. Also, if there is still residual disease, confined to the cervix, at three months after both external and intracavitary radiotherapy, hysterectomy may be justified. In these circumstances the surgery will be less radical than when it is used as the main treatment modality, but the combination can still lead to an unacceptable high rate of complications with a large increase in fistula rate.

Post-operative radiotherapy

Post-operative radiotherapy to the pelvis is required when the surgical specimen either shows that the excision of the tumour is incomplete or the resection margins are close to tumour. When the pelvic nodes contain tumour, pelvic radiotherapy leads to a reduction in the rate of pelvic recurrence but no improvement in survival.

Radiotherapy prescription

A typical dose for external radiotherapy, when treating cervical cancer, is 45–50 Gy to the pelvis, given as 1.8 Gy–2.0 Gy fractions daily, 5 days weekly over 4.5–6 weeks. Fractions above 2.0 Gy increase the risk of late radiation damage. An intracavitary insertion is carried out, no later than 2 weeks after the end of external irradiation, as it has been shown that longer delays in treatment adversely affect the chance of cure. The dose to point A, from the intracavitary insertion, using the Manchester technique, is 25–30 Gy to give a total dose of 75–80 Gy to point A. If a higher than standard dose rate is used, then the dose from the intracavitary treatment is reduced, as discussed in pages 194–197. In the presence of persistent bulky disease within the parametria or involved nodes, parametrial boosts may be delivered to give a further 5 Gy to the involved areas, using external radiotherapy.

The doses received by the rectum and bladder from brachytherapy need to be calculated to ensure that these organs do not receive more than two-thirds of the prescribed dose to point A. These estimations must be carried out prior to the insertion of the active sources. The total dose to the bladder and rectum is preferably no more than 65 Gy to a single reference point.

Chemotherapy

Chemotherapy for cancer of the cervix has been used *concurrently* with radiotherapy, prior to surgery or radiotherapy as *neoadjuvant* therapy, and after surgery or radiotherapy as an *adjuvant* therapy. The main role of chemotherapy is in the treatment of recurrent or metastatic cervical cancer.

For concurrent chemotherapy, cisplatin with or without 5-fluoroucail (5FU) is most commonly used. The success of the combination of mitomycin C and 5FU given with radiotherapy for carcinoma of the anal canal, without causing severe late complications, makes this an interesting combination for appraisal in advanced cancer of the cervix.

Neoadjuvant therapy is being given to a variety of advanced squamous cell tumours to try to improve their prognosis. Cisplatin alone or in combination with methotrexate or with methotrexate and bleomycin has been used in this way for cervical cancer. Ifosfamide, an alkylating agent, is also active. Varying reports have been published in regard to treatment given prior to radiotherapy for advanced cervical disease, and prior to surgery in bulky stage Ib2 tumours. Most published results have shown no advantage for the addition of chemotherapy (e.g. Tattersall *et al.* 1992), but a few have shown benefit, such as the study by Sardi *et al.* (1996). In this latter study, patients with stage IIIb squamous carcinoma were randomized into three groups, of which two received neoadjuvant cisplatin, bleomycin and vincristine prior to pelvic radiotherapy, or surgery and pelvic radiotherapy. Both these groups survived longer compared to the control group that received radiotherapy only.

Post-operative adjuvant chemotherapy is used with or without subsequent radiotherapy in some women where residual disease is suspected or where nodal involvement has been confirmed.

Chemotherapy for recurrent or metastatic carcinoma of the cervix is rarely curative because squamous cell carcinoma of the cervix is not a very chemosensitive tumour. Also, lower response rates are seen in areas which have previously been treated by radiotherapy. The latter is presumably a result of the inability of the drug or drugs to reach the target area because of damage to the microvascular system. It also may be possible that the recurrence after radiotherapy contains clones of cancer cells more resistant to further therapy. However, chemotherapy is a good palliative treatment producing response rates, usually of short duration, in up to 40 percent of patients. The most effective drug, after radiotherapy, is cisplatin at doses of 50–100 mg/m^2 usually given 3-weekly but more frequent scheduling is being investigated.

Novel treatments are being tried for women with advanced or recurrent cervical cancer using new chemotherapeutic agents including the taxanes, gemcitabine, and the topoisomerase-1 inhibitors such as 2-Ironotecan.

Biological agents

Retinoids, for example, *cis*-retinoic acid, which inhibit cell growth and induce cell differentiation, have been reported as being active in cancer of the cervix. Immunological agents, such as the interferons, which also inhibit cell growth and anti-angiogenesis compounds, for example, TNP-470 are all undergoing trials.

NON-SQUAMOUS CARCINOMAS OF THE CERVIX

Adenocarcinoma

Adenocarcinomas arise from the glandular epithelium lining the endo-cervical canal and the endocervical glands.

Adenocarcinoma in situ (ACIS)

Adenocarcinoma *in situ* occurs mainly in women with an average age of around 35 years compared to around 45 years of age for invasive adenocarcinoma. It is much more difficult to define a pre-invasive stage in cervical adenocarcinoma, than in squamous carcinoma, because of the more irregular nature of the basement membrane between the glandular epi-thelium and the underlying stroma. However, pre-invasive forms are being recognized with increasing frequency. It is frequently found in association with CIN.

Invasive adenocarcinoma

Adenocarcinoma of the cervix is becoming more common relative to squamous carcinoma. The incidence has risen from 5 percent of invasive lesions of the cervix to 10–20 percent. This may be a result of a reduction in the incidence of squamous cell carcinoma due to screening (the cervical smear may not be so efficient at detecting endocervical adenocarcinoma) or due to greater awareness by pathologists. The WHO classification divides adenocarcinoma into five histological subtypes: (1) endocervical; (2) endometrioid; (3) adenosquamous; (4) clear cell; and (5) adenoid cystic. One-half to two-thirds of cases are endocervical and up to a quarter are adenosquamous. Serum CEA and CA 125 tumour markers may be raised and many of the tumours are progesterone receptor-positive. The aetiology is less clear than that of squamous carcinoma of the cervix but may be associated with HPV 18.

It is often stated that adenocarcinomas of the cervix has a worse prognosis, stage for stage, than squamous carcinoma. This is probably due to their larger volume at diagnosis as the prognosis appears to be the same for tumours of similar bulk. Adenocarcinomas arise within the endocervical canal and when bulky give rise to a barrel-shaped cervix in which the disease is difficult to eradicate.

Adenosquamous carcinomas in which both elements of squamous and glandular epithelium are malignant, are considered to have a worse prognosis than pure squamous carcinomas of the cervix. Clear cell carcinomas are rare and are mainly found in women whose mothers took diethyl-stilboestrol during pregnancy. Adenoid cystic tumours are extremely rare and generally have a very poor prognosis due to their high incidence of metastatic disease at presentation.

Treatment

Adenocarcinoma in situ *(ACIS)*

Treatment for this lesion is controversial. Conservative treatment with a cone biopsy (either LLETZ or cold knife) completely excising the lesion, may be suitable for women wanting to preserve their child-bearing potential. However, as the adenocarcinoma *in situ* may represent a field change in the whole of the endocervical canal, hysterectomy may be the more appropriate treatment. Colposcopic evaluation is of limited use because the lesion can extend the whole length of the cervical canal.

Invasive disease

The treatment for adenocarcinoma of the cervix is the same as for squamous carcinoma of the cervix. Where radiotherapy is the treatment of choice, total hysterectomy following external radiotherapy has been recommended but the results, compared to radiotherapy alone, have not shown any benefit from this approach.

Verrucous carcinoma of the cervix

Verrucous carcinoma of the cervix is a rare variant of squamous carcinoma. Histologically, they are very similar to condylomata accuminata. They invade locally but rarely metastasize to the lymphatic system.

The treatment is radical hysterectomy, as the tumour is often at an early stage at presentation.

Small cell cancers of the cervix

Small cell carcinomas of the cervix are rare. They can occur as several variants: neuroendocrine, characterized by the presence of neurosecretory granules; carcinoid, arising from argyrophilic cells; oat cell tumours and small cell tumours without neuroendocrine granules or argyrophilic staining. This latter group behaves in a similar fashion to other squamous cell tumours and is treated in the same way. The other three variants carry a very poor prognosis. Treatment is with a combination of surgery, platinum-based chemotherapy and radiotherapy.

Other rare tumours

Malignant lymphomas occasionally occur and, if localized, are treated with radiotherapy or, if more extensive, by chemotherapy which may be followed by radiotherapy to the site of bulk disease. The prognosis is good. Cervical sarcomas and melanomas do poorly.

Special problems

Incidental finding of cervical cancer

Unsuspected invasive cancer of the cervix is occasionally found in women who have had a simple hysterectomy for benign disease or for intra-epithelial neoplasia. The options for treatment are radical surgery or radiotherapy. The radical surgery includes removing the parametrium, upper third of the vagina and the pelvic lymph nodes. Radiation is to the pelvis, to include the pelvic nodes, with a boost to the vaginal vault. The technique and the doses of radiation delivered are similar to those given as an adjuvant for carcinoma of the endometrium (see Chapter 4, p. 88).

The prognosis is good in those cases where there is no residual disease (i.e. small volume tumours) following simple hysterectomy, whether this is followed by further surgery or radiotherapy. If there is significant residual disease following the initial surgery, the outcome is poor regardless of treatment modality.

Cervical cancer during pregnancy

Infrequently, carcinoma of the cervix is discovered during pregnancy. The management will depend on the gestation of the pregnancy, the wishes of the parents, and the stage of disease.

Treatment is similar to that of non-pregnant patients. In the first and second trimester, a Wertheim's hysterectomy is performed for early stage disease and radiotherapy for advanced disease. Between 20 and 28 weeks gestation, it may be possible to wait until fetal maturity develops before proceeding with treatment. As vaginal delivery through the cancer is thought to disseminate the disease a Caesarean Wertheim's operation would be the treatment of choice for early stage disease with appropriate neonatal support for the premature baby. A *classical* Caesarean section is performed delivering the baby through the upper part of the uterus avoiding the cervix. For those patients requiring radiotherapy, hysterotomy, or a classical Caesarean section if the fetus is viable, is carried out prior to the commencement of treatment. Cancer of the cervix suspected during labour should be managed by an emergency Caesarean section.

The 5-year survival of pregnant women with cancer of the cervix is the same, stage for stage, as for the non-pregnant woman.

Haemorrhage

Sometimes carcinoma of the cervix presents with massive haemorrhage. This is usually caused by large exophytic lesions and is treated by vaginal packing under general anaesthesia, bed rest, and blood transfusion. Urgent external beam therapy usually produces haemostasis within 24–48 hours with doses of around 3Gy daily, given for 2–3 days, before continuing with conventional daily dosage. Some radiotherapists prefer to use intracavitary radiotherapy. On rare occasions, ligation of the anterior division of the internal iliac artery or embolization is needed for intractable haemorrhage. (See also Chapter 11, p. 249 on palliation of gynaecological malignancy.)

Recurrence

Eight percent of recurrences from cervical cancer occur within the first two years following treatment. Treatment for recurrence is seldom curative.

Recurrence following radical surgery can be treated by radiotherapy and occasionally long-term remission and apparent cure is achieved. However, the combination of the two treatment modalities, surgery and radiotherapy, can result in severe late radiation effects, especially of the bowel.

Following radical radiotherapy, if the recurrence is central and mobile, radical surgery or exenteration may offer cure. Exenteration is usually necessary as clearance of central recurrence leads to compromise of the irradiated organs. Anterior exenteration includes removal of the bladder, posterior exenteration includes removal of the rectum, and total exenteration includes clearance of all the pelvic contents. The latter results in diversion of both gastrointestinal and urinary tracts but with modern surgery the move is towards pelvic continent reconstruction and away from incontinent stomas (see Chapter 8, p. 167).

Inoperable, recurrent carcinoma of the cervix within an irradiated area may be treated with chemotherapy as discussed previously. As chemotherapy is palliative, it is important to consider the toxicity of treatment in designing a regimen for the patient.

Results

The results reported from FIGO (1988) are shown in Table 3.4 Overall, approximately 50 percent of patients with cancer of the cervix will survive for 5 years. Whilst the 5-year survival for stage I is 76 percent, this rises to over 90 percent for patients with small tumours with uninvolved nodes. As the majority of recurrences (80 percent) from cervical cancer occur in the first 2 years of treatment, 5-year survival rates are a good measure of the effectiveness of treatment of cervical cancer.

The 5-year survival figures are poor for later stage disease due to failure to eradicate bulky disease in the pelvis, rather than to metastatic disease. Local failure rates are approximately 43–52 percent in stage III and 70 percent in stage IVa (Table 3.7). An increase in radiation dose reduces the incidence of pelvic failure with a concomitant increase in complications.

Table 3.7 Incidence of pelvic failure and distant metastases following radiotherapy

Stage	Pelvic failure (%)	Distant metastases (%)
Ib	6–11	7
IIa	7–17	15
IIb	17–30	
IIIb	43–52	29
IVa	70	

Modified from Kim, R. Y. (1993). Radiotherapeutic management in carcinoma of the cervix: current status. *International Journal of Cancer*, 3, 337–48.

Conclusions

An increasing incidence of pre-invasive neoplasia in young women is being detected by screening and is successfully treated. The mortality from cervical cancer in the UK appears to be falling which may be a consequence of screening. However, cervical cancer remains a common cause of death in developing countries.

Both radiotherapy and surgery are equally effective treatments for non-bulky stage I disease, but radiotherapy is the treatment of choice for advanced tumours. Intensification of treatment for advanced disease by the addition of chemotherapy is still being assessed.

References

Austoker, J. (1994). Cancer prevention in primary care. Screening for cervical cancer. *British Medical Journal*, 309, 241–8.

Barton, S. E., Maddox, P. H., Jenkins, D. *et al.* (1988). Effect of cigarette smoking on cervical epithelial immunity: a mechanism for neoplastic change? *Lancet*, 2, 652–4.

Brinton, L. A., Hamman, R. F., Huggins, G. R. *et al.* (1987). Sexual and reproductive risk factors for invasive squamous cell cervical cancer. Journal of the National Cancer Institute, 79, 23–31.

Cuzick, J., Terry, F., Ho, L. *et al.* (1992). Human papilloma virus type 16 DNA in cervical smears as predictor of high-grade cervical cancer. *Lancet*, 339, 959–60.

Hellberg, D. and Nilsson, S. (1989). Genital cancer among wives of men with penile cancer. *British Journal of Obstetrics and Gynaecology*, 96, 221–5.

Irwin, K. L., Rosero-Bixby, L., Oberle, M. W. *et al.* (1988). Oral contraception and cervical cancer risk in Costa Rica. *Journal of the American Medical Association*, 259, 59–64.

Lammont, D. W., Symonds, R. P., Brodie, M. M. *et al.* (1993). Age, socio-economic status and survival from cancer of the cervix in the West of Scotland. *British Journal of Cancer*, 67, 351–35.

Lehtinen, M., Dillner, J., Knept, P. *et al.* (1996). Serologically diagnosed infection with human papillomavirus type 16 and risk for subsequent development of cervical cancer: nested case-control study. *British Medical Journal*, 312, 537–9.

Munoz, N., Bosch, X. and Kaldor, J. M. (1988). Does human papilloma virus cause cervical cancer? The state of the epidemiological evidence. *British Journal of Cancer*, 57, 1–5.

Sardi, J., Giaroli, A., Sananes, C. *et al.* (1996). Randomized trial with neoadjuvant chemotherapy in stage III B squamous carcinoma cervix uteri: an unexpected therapeutic management. *International Journal of Gynecological Cancer*, 6, 85–93.

Sirgurdsson, K. (1993). Effect of organised screening on the risk of cervical cancer. Evaluation of screening activity in Iceland, 1964–1991. *International Journal of Cancer*, 54, 563–70.

Tattersall, M. Ramirez, C., Dalrymple, C. *et al.* (1992). A randomized trial comparing cisplating based chemotherapy followed by radiotherapy vs. radiotherapy alone in patients with Stage IIb–IVa cervical cancer. *International Journal of Gynecological Cancer*, 2, 244–8.

4

Tumours of the uterus

CANCER OF THE ENDOMETRIUM

Incidence

World-wide, there is a high incidence of cancer of the endometrium in white populations in Western Europe and North America but a low rate in Asian populations. It is the most common gynaecological cancer in the USA, but in England and Wales its incidence is lower than that of cancer of the cervix or ovary. Cancer of the endometrium is primarily a disease of postmenopausal women with most occurring in the sixth and seventh decades. In 1988, out of 3789 women diagnosed with this cancer, 92 percent were aged 50 years or older (Table 1.1, p. 4). Less than 5 percent of women are under 40 years of age at the time of diagnosis. The lifetime risk of developing carcinoma of the endometrium is 1.1 percent and the lifetime risk of dying from the tumour is 0.4 percent reflecting its relatively good prognosis (Beral 1995). This good prognosis is because most endometrial cancers are diagnosed at an early stage, when still confined to the body of the uterus. The mortality rate, 30 percent, compares with 50 percent for carcinoma of the cervix and 85 percent for carcinoma of the ovary.

Aetiology

Most of the risk factors for developing endometrial cancer, menarche before age 12 years, delayed menopause after the age of 52 years, infertility, obesity, continuous anovulation as in polycystic ovarian disease, and oestrogen therapy, share the common basis of excessive oestrogen stimulation of the endometrium without the opposing effects of progestogens. An important source of extra-ovarian oestrogens in postmenopausal women is from the aromatization of androgens, produced by the adrenal gland, in fat tissue. The greater the body weight, the greater the peripheral conversion of androgens into oestrogens and thus the higher the blood oestrogen concentration. Consequently, it is not surprising that carcinoma of the endometrium is more common in obese postmenopausal women.

Endometrial hyperplasia, in which there is a proliferation of the endometrial glands and, to a lesser extent, of the endometrial stroma, is thought to be due to unopposed oestrogen stimulation of the endometrium. It may progress to well-differentiated endometrial carcinoma. Hyperplasia can be simple, complex, or atypical. While the first two have a low malignant potential (1–3 percent), atypical hyperplasia has a 23 percent risk of developing into invasive cancer over a period of 11 years (Baker 1996).

The granulosa-theca cell tumour, a rare sex cord stromal tumour of the ovary, can be a source of endogenous oestrogen. Many of these tumours are associated with hyperplasia of the endometrium and endometrial carcinoma occurs in approximately 10 percent of cases. Endometrioid carcinomas of the ovary can also be coincidentally associated with endometrial carcinomas. The endometrial cancers appear to be second primary tumours rather than ovarian metastases. One hypothesis, in regard to this association, is that oestrogen stimulation results in the simultaneous development of both tumours.

Unopposed *exogenous* oestrogens increase the risk of endometrial cancer. This was particularly so in the USA in the 1970s, where hormone replacement therapy (HRT) with oestrogen alone was given to postmenopausal women. The addition of progesterone to oestrogen for 12–14 days of each month's therapy removed this risk and progestogens are now routinely prescribed, with oestrogens, for postmenopausal women requiring HRT and who have not had a hysterectomy. Those that have, can be safely treated with oestrogens alone. It should be noted that women who have previously received pelvic radiotherapy (e.g. for cancer of the cervix) may still have some viable endometrial tissue remaining and therefore require HRT with both oestrogens and progestogens.

The anti-oestrogen, tamoxifen, which is widely used in the treatment of breast cancer has weak oestrogenic effects on the female genital tract. Patients receiving tamoxifen need to be closely monitored for symptoms of abnormal bleeding or discharge, as they have an increased risk of developing endometrial changes including hyperplasia, polyps, and cancer. Seoud *et al.* (1993) reported a twofold increase in the incidence of endometrial cancer in patients receiving tamoxifen over a prolonged period, that is, five years or more.

These are some endometrial tumours that do not appear to be related to oestrogen stimulation. These tumours tend to be poorly differentiated and have a poor prognosis.

Anatomy

The body of the uterus is a pear-shaped, hollow, muscular organ that is in continuity with the fallopian tubes at the cornua superiorly and with the cervix and vagina inferiorly (Fig. 4.1). The widest part of the uterine cavity

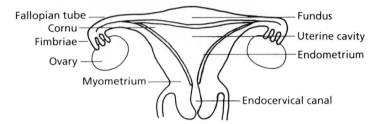

Fig. 4.1 Anatomy of the uterus: the body of the uterus in relation to other gynaecological organs.

is at the fundus (5 cm), which lies between the ostia of the two fallopian tubes. The length of the cavity is approximately 5 cm.

The uterine body is covered externally by peritoneum that is continuous with the broad ligaments laterally. These two folds of peritoneum contain the fallopian tubes and are attached to the ovary by the mesovarium. Inferiorly, the body of the uterus becomes the cervix at the internal os. The parametria on either side of the upper part of the cervix are thickened to form the cardinal ligaments that run to the pelvic side wall and, with the uterosacral ligaments posteriorly, support the uterus (see Fig. 3.3, p. 49). The wall of the uterus is composed of smooth muscle, the myometrium. The cavity is lined by glandular epithelium which is cuboidal before puberty and atrophic after the menopause. In the reproductive years, the glandular elements are under the influence of the ovarian hormones, oestrogens and progestogens, which are controlled by the pituitary gonadotrophins, follicle stimulating hormone (FSH) and luteinizing hormone (LH). Oestrogen produces proliferation of the endometrium before ovulation and, with the added effect of progestogen, a secretory phase after ovulation. Unless pregnancy occurs, the endometrium is shed monthly—the menses.

The lymphatic drainage is to the pelvic and para-aortic nodes (Fig. 4.2).

Spread of disease

Cancer of the endometrium can spread directly through the endometrial cavity to the cervix and along the fallopian tubes to the ovaries and peritoneal cavity. Tumour frequently infiltrates the myometrium and can extend to the serosal surface of the uterus or into the parametria. Very advanced cases of endometrial cancer may resemble advanced ovarian cancer with widespread intra-abdominal metastases. Very rarely, there is direct invasion of the pubic bones.

Spread via the lymphatic system is to both the pelvic and para-aortic nodes with pelvic node metastases being more common. Involvement of the para-aortic nodes may occur directly via lymphatics from the upper part of

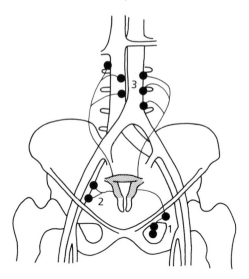

Fig. 4.2 The lymph node drainage of the uterus: (1) inguinal nodes; (2) pelvic nodes; (3) para-aortic nodes.

the uterus draining to the fallopian tube and ovary but it is more usual for para-aortic nodes to be involved in the presence of pelvic lymphadenopathy. Very rarely, lymphatic spread occurs to the inguinal nodes. Blood-borne spread is uncommon and is usually to the lungs.

Pathology

Adenocarcinomas arise from the glandular elements of the endometrium. Most endometrial carcinomas arise in the upper region of the uterus, often as a raised or papillary area. The internal os is not usually involved until the disease becomes extensive within the uterus *Endometrioid* adenocarcinoma is the commonest type of adenocarcinoma, accounting for approximately 90 percent of all cases. Benign squamous changes are present in 20–25 percent of such tumours. These latter tumours are known as *adeno-acanthomas*, but their behaviour and prognosis is no different from that of a pure endometrioid adenocarcinoma. Rarely, the squamous element is malignant (*adenosquamous carcinomas*).

Other histological types of tumour of the endometrium are rare. *Papillary serous* carcinoma behaves in a similar fashion to ovarian serous papillary carcinoma and has a poor prognosis. *Clear cell* carcinoma resembles renal clear cell carcinoma but has its origin in Mullerian structures. It also has a poor prognosis. Extremely rare is *squamous* carcinoma in which a cervical primary must first be excluded. *Metastatic spread* may be directly from another pelvic malignancy or rarely from a distant site such as the breast.

Screening

Unlike cancer of the cervix, there is no cost-effective screening test available for endometrial cancer in asymptomatic women. Most endometrial cancers present at an early stage, usually with abnormal vaginal bleeding and, in particular, postmenopausal bleeding. Any woman over the age of 40 years with abnormal bleeding must be considered at risk of endometrial cancer and requires investigation to exclude an underlying malignant cause before being treated for a benign condition.

Symptoms and signs

As stated above, the most common presenting symptom of endometrial cancer is abnormal vaginal bleeding (postmenopausal, intermenstrual, post-coital bleeding, or altered menstrual pattern). As the majority of women with endometrial cancer are over 50 years of age, about 75 percent will present with postmenopausal bleeding. While the causes of postmenopausal bleeding are numerous, there is a 10–20 percent risk of endometrial cancer, particularly with increasing age. In younger women, the abnormal bleeding is usually intermenstrual but over one-third of premenopausal women with endometrial cancer complain of regular but heavy menses.

Rarely, the presenting symptom is pain which indicates advanced or metastatic disease. Vaginal discharge may occur which may be tumour-related or due to infection within the uterine cavity—a pyometra. The presence of a pyometra in a postmenopausal woman should alert the clinician to a possible underlying malignancy. Rarely, bleeding into the uterine cavity from an endometrial malignancy, in the presence of a blocked endocervical canal, will lead to a haematometra.

A complete clinical assessment is needed including both a rectal and a vaginal examination. There is often an absence of clinical signs but the uterus may feel enlarged and blood may be seen in the vagina.

Investigations

In view of the usual presenting symptom of abnormal vaginal bleeding, the most important initial tests are a transvaginal scan (TVS) and outpatient endometrial biopsy (e.g. using a Pipelle). A transvaginal ultrasound exam-ination measures the endometrial thickness and views the ovaries. In the postmenopausal group, if a scan shows normal ovaries and thin endo-metrium (5 mm or less) and the endometrial biopsy is benign, then no further action is necessary. If, however, the endometrium is thickened on transvaginal scan, which is suggestive of pathology, or there is insufficient material from the endometrial biopsy for diagnosis, then a hysteroscopy followed by a D&C (dilatation and curettage) is carried out. The theoretical advantage of hysteroscopy is that it allows visualization of the complete cavity enabling direct biopsy of suspicious areas but it is not always possible to distinguish abnormal endometrium. There is no added advantage to performing a fractional curettage (samples taken from the endocervix and then from the body of the uterus) as it offers no extra reliable information. Hysteroscopy and D&C, performed under general anaesthetic, can be carried out as a day case or overnight stay.

Routine investigations include chest X-ray, intravenous urography, or ultrasonography to examine the renal tract, blood indices, renal and liver function tests. In addition, pre-operative staging can be carried out using magnetic resonance imaging (MRI) to determine the depth of myometrial invasion and the presence of lymphadenopathy. Ultrasound can also be used to assess myometrial invasion.

Staging

The staging of endometrial cancer is performed according to the FIGO classification (Table 4.1). Although a full surgico-pathological staging is

Table 4.1 Modified FIGO staging for carcinoma of the endometrium

Stage	Features
I	Confined to the corpus
Ia	Carcinoma confined to the endometrium
Ib	Myometrial invasion <50%
Ic	Myometrial invasion >50%
II	Cervix involved
IIa	Endocervical gland involvement only
IIb	Cervical stromal invasion but does not extend beyond the uterus
III	
IIIa	Carcinoma involves serosa of uterus or adnexae, or positive ascites/or positive peritoneal washings
IIIb	Vaginal involvement either direct or metastatic
IIIc	Para-aortic or pelvic node involvement
IV	
IVa	Carcinoma involving the mucosa of the bladder or rectum
IVb	Distant metastases and involvement of other abdominal or inguinal lymph nodes

FIGO, International Federation of Gynaecology and Obstetrics.

recommended by FIGO, the majority of women in the UK do not have a lymphadenectomy performed. There is some evidence to suggest that lymphadenectomy may lead to improved survival (Kilgore *et al.* 1995), although it is accepted that not all women will be fit enough for the additional surgery.

For each stage the degree of differentiation, grade 1 (well differentiated), grade 2 (moderately differentiated), or grade 3 (poorly differentiated), is also recorded. For grade 1, there must be 5 percent or less of a non-squamous solid growth pattern, that is, no glands are present; grade 2, 6–50 percent of a non-squamous solid growth pattern; grade 3, more than 50 percent of a non-squamous solid growth pattern. In addition, if there is notable nuclear atypia inappropriate for grades 1 or 2, the grade is raised to the next grade. Adenocarcinomas with squamous differentiation are graded according to the nuclear grade of the glandular component and in serous, clear cell adenocarcinomas, and squamous cell carcinomas, nuclear grading takes precedence.

Prognostic factors

Many prognostic factors have been identified for endometrial cancer, of which the most important are stage of disease, depth of myometrial invasion and tumour grade which closely correlate with lymph node status. Other factors include age at diagnosis, body morphology, type and size of tumour, lymphovascular space involvement, steroid receptor status, ploidy, and overexpression of oncogenes.

Stage

The survival rates for the different stages of endometrial cancer are shown on Table 4.2. The overall survival for endometrial cancer is high as there is a preponderance of women diagnosed with stage I disease, however, stage for stage, the survival rates are similar to those for cancer of the cervix.

Staging reflects tumour volume, which is related to the risk of pelvic and para-aortic node involvement. The greater the tumour volume, the higher

Table 4.2 Five-year survival by stage (modified from FIGO 1988)

Stage	% of total	5-year survival (%)
I	74	72
II	13.5	56
III	6	31.5
IV	3	10.5

the risk and the poorer the prognosis. Even within stage 1, tumour size is of significance. Schink *et al.* (1991) found, in a study on 91 patients with stage I disease, that patients with small lesions (less than 2 cm diameter) had a 4 percent incidence of lymph node metastases compared to 15 percent when the tumour was greater than 2 cm, increasing to 35 percent when the entire endometrium was involved.

Stage II indicates that the endometrial carcinoma is involving the endocervix. This correlates with a poorer prognosis as there is a twofold increase in lymph node metastasis—20 percent compared to 10 percent (Table 4.3). Once the adnexa are involved (stage IIIa) the pelvic nodal metastatic rate rises to 52% (COSA-NZ-UK Endometrial Cancer Study Groups 1996).

Depth of myometrial invasion

Myometrial invasion is reflected in the staging for stage I endometrial carcinoma (Table 4.1; Fig. 4.3) and the depth of invasion is a good indicator of spread to the pelvic and para-aortic lymph nodes in early carcinoma of the endometrium (Table 4.3). There is close correlation between tumour grade and depth of myometrial invasion (Table 4.4) with the depth of inva-

Table 4.3 Incidence of positive lymph nodes (pelvic and para-aortic) in patients with stage I and II endometrial carcinoma relating to depth of myometrial invasion[a]

Myometrial invasion	No. of patients	% with nodal involvement
None	105	2
<1/3	446	7
Mid 1/3	229	5
>2/3	234	24
All stage I	1014	10
All stage II	93	20

[a] Summary of three lymphadenectomy series (COSA-NZ-UK Endometrial Cancer Study Group 1996; Creasman *et al.* 1987; Calais *et al.* 1990).
Table modified from Thomas and Blake (1996).

Table 4.4 Correlation of tumour grade with depth of myometrial invasion (expressed as a percentage)

| Myometrial invasion | FIGO grade | | |
	1	2	3
No invasion (%)	58	52	38
<1/2 myometrial invasion (%)	30	28	16
>1/2 myometrial invasion (%)	12	20	46

From Boronow (1985); Creasman *et al.* (1987).

sion being the more important predictor. Grade 1 tumours are usually associ-ated with only superficial invasion but even well-differentiated tumours, when deeply invasive, are more likely to have spread to the lymph nodes, resulting in a poorer prognosis.

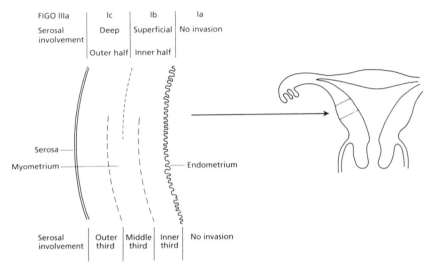

Fig. 4.3 Diagram of a section of the wall of the uterus showing the two commonly used measurements of depth of myometrial invasion in either halves (FIGO) or thirds.

Tumour grade

As the tumour becomes less differentiated, the risk of deep myometrial involvement with associated lymph node involvement increases (Table 4.5). Almost 90 percent of grade 1 tumours will be limited to the endometrium (stage Ia) or inner half of the myometrium (stage Ib) while almost half of those with grade 3 histology will invade the outer half of the myometrium

Table 4.5 Incidence of positive lymph nodes (pelvic and para-aortic) in patients with stage I and II endometrial carcinoma according to grade[a]

Grade	No. of patients	Nodal involvement (%)
1	297	6
2	439	9
3	278	16

[a] Summary of three lymphadenectomy series (COSA-NZ-UK Endometrial Cancer Study Group 1996; Creasman *et al.* 1987; Calais *et al.* 1990.
Table modified from Thomas and Blake (1996).

Table 4.6 Five-year disease-free survival for surgical
stage I endometrial carcinoma (expressed as a
percentage) (From Grigsby 1992)

Myometrial invasion	FIGO grade		
	1	2	3
No invasion (%)	96	92	85
<1/2 myometrial invasion (%)	95	90	69
>1/2 myometrial invasion (%)	81	70	42

(stage Ic) (Table 4.4). As a consequence, survival for patients with stage I
endometrial cancer is also dependant on the grade of tumour (Table 4.6).
The majority of cases of stage I disease are grade 1 or 2 and only about 20
percent are grade 3.

Rare endometrial adenocarcinomas

The rare tumour types of endometrial carcinoma, serous papillary, clear
cell, and squamous carcinoma all have a poor prognosis. The overall
survival for these carcinomas is less than 33 percent (Wilson *et al.* 1990).

Lymph node involvement

The higher incidence of lymph node involvement with increasing stage, has
already been discussed. In *clinical* stage I disease, the incidence of *surgical*
lymph node involvement, both pelvic and para-aortic was examined by the
GOG in a study of 621 patients (Creasman *et al.* 1987). Overall, 9 percent
of patients were found to have involvement of pelvic lymph nodes and
6 percent para-aortic node involvement. The incidence of para-aortic
node involvement *without* coexisting pelvic node involvement was only 2
percent.

In this study, nodal metastases were found to be associated with grade 3
histology, deep myometrial invasion, involvement of the cervix or lower
segment of the uterus, adnexal or extra-uterine involvement, lymphovascular space involvement, positive peritoneal cytology, and histological
types other than endometrioid adenocarcinoma. Later studies of nodal
involvement showed similar findings in patients treated by pelvic lymphadenectomy by Calais *et al.* (1990) and by the COSA-NZ-UK Endometrial
Study Group (1996). The data has been combined to show the incidence of
positive pelvic nodes in relation to both depth of myometrial invasion and
grade in stages I and II endometrial cancer in Tables 4.3 and 4.5.

Lymphovascular space involvement

Lymphovascular space involvement appears to be an important prognostic
indicator for stage I endometrial cancer. A recent study (Gal *et al.* 1996)

showed lymphovascular space involvement to be an important independent indicator for both recurrence and survival.

Peritoneal cytology

The significance of positive peritoneal cytology as a prognostic sign in endometrial cancer remains unresolved as it is usually only found in the presence of other poor prognostic signs (Lurain 1992).

Steroid receptors

Receptors for both oestrogen and progesterone are present in approximately 70 percent of endometrial carcinomas. Tumours that are receptor-negative or have a low number of receptors have a worse prognosis. Advanced stage disease with poor differentiation, clear cell, and serous papillary tumours are all more likely to be receptor negative.

Ploidy

DNA ploidy and the fraction of cells in the S phase are prognostic factors which correlate strongly with stage and tumour grade. Most endometrial cancers are diploid but aneuploidy indicates advanced disease and a poor prognosis. A raised fraction of cells in the S phase also indicates a poorer prognosis.

Growth factors

The overexpression of growth factors in endometrial cancer is discussed in Chapter 7, on molecular biology.

Age and body morphology

Older women have a worse prognosis than younger women. This is partly, but not wholly, due to their higher incidence of poorly differentiated and deeply invasive tumours. Obese patients with a high level of endogenous oestrogens, tend to have superficial and well-differentiated cancers and, therefore, have a good prognosis.

Treatment

Surgery

The primary treatment of patients with clinical stage I endometrial cancer is total hysterectomy and bilateral salpingo-oophorectomy. FIGO staging requires the status of the peritoneal cytology (easily obtained at operation without extra morbidity) and the pelvic and para-aortic lymph nodes to be assessed. However, in the UK, a pelvic and para-aortic lymphadenectomy is usually not performed by the general gynaecologist. In the USA, hysterectomy with pelvic and para-aortic lymphadenectomy is performed either at open operation or via laparoscopy.

As patients with *pathological* stage II and stage IIIa cancer of the endometrium are diagnosed post-operatively their surgical treatment is the same as for those patients with stage I disease. Women with *clinical* stage II cancer of the endometrium are treated as if they have stage I cancer of the cervix (i.e. with a radical hysterectomy or radical radiotherapy). It may not be clear whether the cervical involvement is due to an endometrial cancer spreading down into the cervix or an endocervical cancer spreading upwards into the uterus. For patients with clinical stage III or IV disease radiotherapy, with or without hormonal treatment and chemotherapy, is the standard mode of therapy. Rarely, as a palliative procedure, limited surgery to remove the central tumour is carried out.

Radiotherapy

Radiotherapy is given as:

(1) an adjunct to surgery;

(2) radical treatment; and

(3) palliation.

Adjuvant radiotherapy for stage I cancer

The need for radiotherapy as an adjuvant to surgery in stage I carcinoma of the endometrium is unclear. Pre-operative radiotherapy has been replaced by appropriate post-operative radiotherapy as this allows full assessment of the pathology before deciding on the necessity for further treatment. The indications for post-operative radiotherapy vary between clinicians but a decision will be based on the known risks of pelvic or vaginal vault recurrence and of pelvic node involvement.

For early stage endometrial carcinoma some radiotherapists give vaginal vault irradiation to prevent vault recurrence. All patients are treated except for those whose tumours show either no or only minimal myometrial invasion, are in the upper part of the uterus and are grades 1 or 2 histology. However, the Danish Endometrial Cancer Group, who gave no post-operative radiotherapy to 641 patients with stage I 'low-risk' disease (stage Ia and b, grade 1 and 2) had a recurrence rate of only 7 percent at five years. The group concluded that radiotherapy was not indicated in these low-risk cases (Poulsen *et al.* 1996).

The dose of radiotherapy with intracavitary therapy to the vaginal vault is typically 60 Gy, measured at the surface of the applicator, or its equivalent with high dose rate therapy (36 Gy in 6 fractions in 3 weeks). This is given using either ovoids or a vaginal obturator. Some radiotherapists treat the whole vagina in order to prevent lower vaginal as well as vault recurrence.

The indication for giving external beam therapy irradiation to the pelvis depends on whether there is adnexal involvement or a high likelihood of spread having occurred to the pelvic nodes. The tumour characteristics that indicate possible nodal involvement and therefore a worse prognosis have already been listed (p. 82). They include lower uterine segment or cervical involvement, deep myometrial penetration, and poor differentiation (grade 3) of the tumour. There is little evidence that postoperative external beam radiotherapy increases survival in this poor prognostic group by preventing metastases, but it does reduce the local pelvic recurrence rate especially in poorly differentiated adenocarcinomas (Aalders *et al.* 1980). Usually, vault radiotherapy is given at the end of external beam therapy but the necessity for this additional radiotherapy is unproven.

A suggested post-operative radiotherapy protocol for stage I disease is shown on Table 4.7. A typical dose to the pelvis for the treatment of occult nodal metastases is 45 Gy given in 25 fractions over 5 weeks with a further 20–25 Gy to the vaginal mucosa (or 12 Gy in 2 fractions using high dose rate) given by intracavitary brachytherapy. The pelvis is treated as for cancer of the cervix but to the bottom of L5 vertebra. Para-aortic nodes are not normally treated prophylactically because of increased morbidity and lack of evidence for any survival benefit.

Pelvic lymphadenectomy or post-operative radiotherapy for stage I?

Pelvic lymphadenectomy is an alternative to post-operative radiotherapy for those patients in whom it is considered necessary to treat the pelvic nodes. The arguments for and against lymphadenectomy have been reviewed by Thomas and Blake (1996), who concluded that there was no reason for the current policy of limited surgery followed by adjuvant radiotherapy when indicated, to be changed until randomized studies have been carried out.

The COSA-NZ-UK Endometrial Cancer Study Groups (1996) reviewed 238 patients with 'high-risk' endometrial cancer (grade 3 endometrioid,

Table 4.7 Suggested post-operative radiotherapy protocol for stage I endometrial carcinoma

Myometrial invasion	FIGO grade	Treatment
No invasion	1 and 2	None unless tumour in lower uterine segment: if so, vaginal irradiation
<1/2 myometrial invasion	1 and 2	Vaginal irradiation only
>1/2 myometrial invasion (vaginal)	1 and 2	External beam pelvic irradiation plus irradiation
All depths	3; *or* lymphvascular invasion or tumour in lower uterine segment	External beam pelvic irradiation plus vaginal irradiation

adenosquamous, clear cell or serous papillary histology, depth of myometrial invasion more than one-third, cervical or adnexal involvement) treated by hysterectomy and pelvic lymphadenectomy. The patients chosen for this extended surgery were younger and less obese than women treated with hysterectomy and bilateral salpingo-oophorectomy (BSO), followed by external and vault radiotherapy. If positive nodes were found at lymphadenectomy, pelvic and vaginal radiotherapy was given post-operatively but, if the nodes were negative, only the vaginal vault was irradiated. The results showed that patients who had a lymphadenectomy had a similar cancer-free survival to those treated by simple surgery with adjuvant radiotherapy alone. These findings suggested that hysterectomy and pelvic lymphadenectomy is a reasonable alternative to hysterectomy and post-operative pelvic radiotherapy, in younger and fitter patients with high-risk disease. However, there is no data on the morbidity that resulted from this approach.

The disadvantages of selective pelvic lymphadenectomy have to be balanced against the disadvantages of pelvic radiotherapy. First, many patients with endometrial cancer would not tolerate this more extensive surgery in view of risk factors such as advanced age, obesity, hypertension, and diabetes mellitus. Second, as accurate identification of those patients who might benefit from extended surgery is not easy this could result in unnecessary lymphadenectomies.

There is also controversy concerning the increased risks of complications with more extensive surgery, with or without adjuvant radiotherapy. Some studies (Bablionti 1989; Holmesley *et al.* 1992) showing no increased morbidity while Calais *et al.* (1990) reporting an immediate post-operative complication rate of 17 percent. Randomized studies are being established in the UK to compare hysterectomy alone with hysterectomy and pelvic lymphadenectomy.

Radiotherapy for stage II cancer

The majority of women with stage II disease are diagnosed on examination of the pathological specimen. These cases are treated with post-operative radiotherapy to the pelvis and vaginal vault as for stage I endometrial cancer. For bulky stage II disease, if radiotherapy is the mode of treatment, some clinicians advise carrying out a total hysterectomy after radiotherapy is completed in order to ensure complete eradication of tumour within the uterus. However, the combination of radical radiotherapy and surgery increases the risk of complications.

Radiotherapy for stage III and IV cancer

Radiotherapy is the standard treatment for stage clinical III cancers of the endometrium which occur in less than 10 percent of recorded cases. In those patients with stage IIIa, where there is only a microscopic deposit in the fallopian tubes or ovaries, the prognosis is good but where the disease is gross, survival is poor.

Post-operative radiotherapy to the pelvis and vaginal vault is given to patients found to have stage III disease at surgery. Treatment is as for stage I but if the vagina is involved, the whole of its length is irradiated. When there is pelvic or para-aortic node involvement (stage IIIc), ascites or positive peritoneal washings, chemotherapy or progestogen therapy may be given in addition to radiotherapy. Irradiation of the para-aortic nodes is seldom justified as the benefit of using an extended field is unproven and would be poorly tolerated by the majority of this group of patients.

In the presence of gross stage III or IV disease treatment is seldom curative. If the patient is fit, chemotherapy is given either before radiotherapy or concurrently to try to improve local control. Radiotherapy for stage IV disease is usually palliative.

Radical radiotherapy

The rare patient with stage I cancer of the endometrium, who is medically unfit for surgery, is treated with radical radiotherapy. As the outcome for radiotherapy alone is poor, every attempt should be made to treat the central tumour surgically.

There are two ways of treating cancer of the endometrium by radiotherapy, one is by intracavitary radiotherapy alone and the second is by external radiotherapy followed by an intracavitary insertion. External radiotherapy is useful in the presence of a large uterine tumour, as it can reduce its size prior to intracavitary treatment, as well as treating the parametria and pelvic nodes. Frequently, however, patients who are unsuitable for surgery are also unsuitable for a prolonged course of external radiotherapy and are therefore treated by intracavitary treatment alone.

Intracavitary therapy   Historically, this was carried out by packing the uterine cavity with Heyman's capsules containing radium-226. This technique is still carried out using afterloading techniques with caesium-137, but in the UK it is more usual to use a long intrauterine tube and ovoids placed in the vaginal vault. A dose of 70–80 Gy to point A (p. 185 and Fig. 9.4) is given in two insertions one week apart, for a low dose rate system. Alternatively, the dose may be prescribed to the serosa of the uterus if this can be imaged on computerized tomographic (CT) scan with the applicators in place. The dose to the serosa would usually be limited to 60–70 Gy in 2 fractions. With high dose rate after-loading systems computerized programmes allow for individualization of treatment so ensuring complete irradiation of the uterine cavity, whatever its size. With the microSelectron, specially curved intrauterine applicators of various lengths can be directed first into one cornua and then the other so that the radiation field completely covers the uterus including the most distant lateral points. However, there is no evidence that these conformal methods of radiotherapy are superior to a central intrauterine tube.

Palliative radiotherapy

Palliative radiotherapy is used for advanced endometrial cancer unsuitable for surgery and for metastatic or recurrent endometrial carcinoma. Treatment will depend on the site of the disease and the medical condition of the patient. It is particularly useful in treating vaginal bleeding and metastatic bony pain.

Complications of radiotherapy and surgery

The complications of treatment are discussed fully in the chapters on surgery and radiotherapy. However, with surgery limited to a total hysterectomy and bilateral salpingo-oopherectomy, followed by radiotherapy using a standard technique, the complication rate should be low.

Hormonal therapy

Progestogens

Progestogens are the most frequently used form of hormone therapy. Their main contribution has been in treating recurrent disease and overall response rates of 15–30 percent have been reported. Medroxyprogesterone acetate is the most commonly prescribed progestogen in doses of 200–400 mg daily. Patients with well-differentiated tumours, which are more likely to have positive oestrogen receptor (ER) or progesterone receptor (PR) status, have a response rate of up to 50 percent. Similarly, late recurrences respond to this therapy more often than recurrences occurring soon after primary treatment, probably related to better tumour differentiation and the increased presence of hormone receptors in more slowly developing tumours. Progestogens have been given prior to surgery to induce tumour differentiation and postoperatively as adjuvant therapy in the absence of residual disease. Most studies have failed to show a benefit from progestogens as adjuvant therapy. Progestogens should therefore not be given unless there is evidence of persistent tumour.

Other hormones

Tamoxifen can increase intracellular progesterone receptor (PR) content, and has been used in advanced and recurrent disease refractory to progestogen therapy, with occasional responses. Higher response rates are seen in patients who have previously responded to progestogens, showing the tumour to be hormone-sensitive. Tamoxifen can also be given to increase PR status prior to giving progestogen therapy, or in combination therapy using both drugs either sequentially or together.

Gonadotrophin releasing hormone (GnRH) analogues lower the concentration of serum luteinizing hormone (LH). Their mode of action is to produce a continuous rather than a pulsed stimulus of the anterior pituitary gonadotrophins, leading to receptor down-regulation. Responses to GnRH analogues (e.g. goserelin and leuprorelin) have been seen in patients with endometrial cancer refractory to progestogen therapy. The drugs can be given as monthly or three-monthly depot injections.

Chemotherapy

Adjuvant chemotherapy is seldom given in endometrial cancer but should be considered in fit patients with systemic disease. In the management of *recurrent* endometrial cancer the role of chemotherapy is often limited because of advanced age and poor performance status. The anthracyclines, doxorubicin and epirubicin, and the platinum drugs, cisplatin and carbo-platin, are all effective drugs used alone or in combination with response rates of 20–35 percent. Responses tend to be partial and of short duration.

Treatment of recurrent and metastatic disease

In those patients in whom surgery was the only mode of treatment for the initial disease radiotherapy can be used for local recurrence within the pelvis. The role of radiotherapy for metastases has already been discussed. Usually, treatment of recurrent and metastatic endometrial cancer is with progestogens, as described above and, in hormone-resistant patients who are fit, chemotherapy may be given with palliative intent.

Results

Endometrial carcinoma is considered to have a good prognosis. This is due to the preponderance of early stage disease and 5-year disease-free survival rates of over 90 percent have been recorded for patients with stage I disease with minimal myometrial invasion or who are found after surgery to have no evidence of nodal involvement (Table 4.6). The 5-year disease-free survival, however, falls to under 60 percent for those with positive pelvic nodes. The 72 percent, 5-year survival figure, for stage I, reported by FIGO (1988, Table 4.2) is not disease-specific and reflects deaths from other causes in an elderly population with medical complications. In advanced disease, which affects less than 10 percent of women with endometrial cancer, the prognosis is as poor as it is for any other advanced gynaeco-logical cancer (Table 4.2).

HRT after endometrial cancer

Although HRT with unopposed oestrogens has been found to be associated with an increased incidence of endometrial cancer in women with an intact uterus, there is no evidence that HRT with oestrogen alone is contra-indicated in women who have undergone radical treatment for early stage endometrial cancer. However, where there is a fear that sugery is incomplete, or that there is residual or metastatic disease, HRT with progestogens alone is indicated, e.g. Medroxyprogesterone Acetate 20–40mg daily.

Conclusions

Carcinoma of the endometrium occurs mainly in postmenopausal women, and oestrogens appear to play a part in its causation. It is usually diagnosed at an early stage as the most common symptom, postmenopausal bleeding, occurs when the cancer is still confined to the body of the uterus.

The primary treatment for endometrial cancer, in the UK at the present time, is total hysterectomy and bilateral salpingo-oophorectomy. This is followed by radiotherapy to the pelvis and/or vaginal vault to reduce the incidence of local recurrence, when the patient is thought to be at increased risk on account of lower uterine or cervical involvement, high histological grade, type of tumour, depth of myometrial penetration more than half the thickness of the myometrium, and lymphovascular space involvement. There is increasing interest in the role of pelvic lymphadenectomy in this high-risk group which would limit the need for post-operative radiotherapy to those women with proven pelvic node metastases. Extended surgery might also lead to better rates of disease-free survival.

Hormonal manipulation can be useful in the management of recurrent disease. There is little evidence for a role for progestogens as adjuvant therapy.

UTERINE SARCOMAS

Introduction

Uterine sarcomas are rare tumours that are usually highly malignant and occur in 2 per 100 000 women. They account for about 4 percent of all uterine cancers. They are normally staged in a similar way to endometrial carcinomas although the substages do not apply to sarcomas. Tumour spread commonly includes haematogenous as well as lymphatic routes. There are several histological classifications. The main types seen are endometrial stromal sarcoma, myometrial tumours, of which by far the commonest is leiomyosarcoma, and malignant mixed mullerian tumours.

Endometrial stromal sarcoma (ESS)

These tumours occur in women aged 40–55 years, a younger age group than for other uterine sarcomas. They are divided into low grade and high grade endometrial stromal sarcoma on the basis of mitotic count and the nature of the infiltrating border.

Low grade endometrial stromal sarcoma

This was previously known as endolymphatic stromal myosis. It arises in the stroma or in areas of adenomyosis or endometriosis. The tumours are usually infiltrating, causing thickening of the uterine wall. Microscopically, the structure resembles normal endometrial stroma with only mild nuclear atypia. Finger-like projections of stromal cells infiltrate between the muscle fibres of the myometrium into lymphatic spaces. Although abnormal vaginal bleeding may occur, the lesion is usually found incidentally at the time of hysterectomy.

These low grade tumours have a tendency to relapse with a recurrence rate of 50 percent in stage I disease. Recurrences, which can occur up to 10 years after initial diagnosis, are mainly within the pelvis but can be found in extra-pelvic sites. Nodal involvement is unusual.

The treatment is surgery, that is, hysterectomy and salpingo-oophorectomy. It is recommended that those women with lesions larger than 5 cm or with parametrial invasion or venous invasion should receive post-operative radiotherapy to the pelvis *or* high dose progestogens such as 1000 mg of medroxyprogesterone acetate daily (Morrow *et al.* 1993). The decision on which treatment should be given depend on whether progesterone receptors are present in the tumour. Radiotherapy and/or progestogen therapy is given for recurrent disease but anthracycline-based chemotherapy should also be considered.

High grade endometrial stromal sarcoma

High grade endometrial stromal sarcoma (ESS) is a highly malignant tumour with a very poor prognosis. It usually presents as a polypoid mass in the uterine cavity which causes vaginal bleeding. Treatment is surgery followed by pelvic radiotherapy, the latter in an attempt to prevent local recurrence. Chemotherapy is indicated for advanced or recurrent disease. Drugs with activity in high grade ESS include doxorubicin, cisplatin, and ifosfamide.

Leiomyosarcomas

Leiomyosarcomas constitute 30–40 percent of all uterine sarcomas but only about 2 percent of all smooth muscle tumours of the uterus are malignant;

the vast majority are benign leiomyomata (fibroids). Only 5–10 percent of leiomyosarcomas arise in an existing fibroid, although they may develop in a fibroid uterus. Most are solitary tumours with a tendency to spread to lymph nodes and to the abdominal cavity. Their macroscopic appearance resembles that of a fibroid, but microscopically the presence of 10 mitoses per 10 high power fields, the presence of coagulative necrosis, nuclear atypia, and an infiltrating invasive front distinguishes sarcomas. Most occur in the sixth decade and postmenopausal bleeding is the usual first symptom. Frequently, the diagnosis is not made until hysterectomy, often carried out for what are thought to be simple fibroids.

Surgical treatment is the same as for ESS but there is no evidence that pelvic radiotherapy will prevent local recurrence. In view of the very high incidence of recurrence of these tumours adjuvant anthracyline-based chemotherapy has been recommended but there are no data to show that this improves the very poor survival rates. Chemotherapy with doxorubicin is the treatment of choice for advanced and recurrent disease.

Mixed mesodermal tumour

Mixed mesodermal tumour is the most common uterine sarcoma, and usually occurs in women aged between 60 and 70 years. As their name suggests, they contain both malignant epithelial and malignant stromal elements in varying proportions, and they have a characteristic histological picture. The epithelial element is usually an endometrioid carcinoma and is poorly differentiated. The stromal element may be *homologous*, that is, composed of malignant cells derived from types that are normally found in the uterus, such as leiomyosarcoma, fibrosarcoma, and endometrial stromal sarcoma, or they may be undifferentiated. Homologous mixed mesodermal tumours are frequently reported as 'carcinosarcomas'. If the elements are not related to normal uterine tissue, as with rhabdomyo-sarcoma, osteosarcoma, and chondrosarcoma, then the tumour is described as *heterologous*.

The tumour, which distends the uterus and is frequently found protruding through the cervical os at diagnosis, usually causes vaginal bleeding and can also cause pressure symptoms from the mass, or pain. Lymphatic spread occurs in a manner similar to poorly differentiated adenocarcinomas of the endometrium and blood-borne metastases to the lungs are not uncommon. Polypoidal lesions with no invasion of the myometrium may occur and these have the best prognosis.

The surgical treatment for mixed mesodermal tumours is similar to other sarcomas. Post-operative radiotherapy to the pelvis is recommended to reduce the likelihood of pelvic recurrence and for advanced or recurrent disease the anthracyclines (e.g. doxorubicin), cisplatin, and ifosfamide have all been shown to have activity.

Adenosarcoma

Adenosarcoma is a mixed mesodermal tumour in which only the stromal element is malignant. It is of low-grade malignancy. Recurrence can occur usually several years after hysterectomy and then further surgery should be considered.

Results

With the exception of low grade ESS, the polypoidal mixed mesodermal tumour with little or no myometrial invasion and the rare leiomyosarcoma occurring within a fibroid, the overall prognosis for uterine sarcomas, regardless of type, is very poor indeed and for practical purposes there are no survivors at five years. Even for stage I, the two-year survival is only 45 percent. Relapse is common in the pelvis, pelvic nodes, abdomen and lungs, and, while pelvic radiotherapy reduces pelvic recurrence in high grade ESS and mixed Mullerian tumours, it does not affect prognosis. Adjuvant chemotherapy has no proven role in increasing survival. For low grade ESS, progestogens are an effective treatment for recurrent disease, resulting in long-term remissions.

References

Aalders, J., Abeler, V., Kolstad, P., and Onstud, M. (1980). Post-operative external, irradiation and prognostic parameters in stage I endometrial carcinoma. *Obstetrics and Gynecology*, 56, 419–27.

Bablionti, L., Di Petro, G., La Fianzo, A. *et al.* (1989). Complications of pelvic lymphadenectomy in patients with endometrial cancer. *European Journal of Gynecological Oncology*, 10, 2–5.

Baker, T. R. (1996). Premalignant conditions of the endometrium (endometrial hyperplasia and adenocarcinoma in situ). In *Handbook of gynecologic oncology* (2nd edn). (ed. M. S. Piver), pp. 133–40. Little Brown and Co, Boston.

Beral, V. (1995). Prevention of cancers of the female genital tract. In *The biology of gynaecological cancer* (ed. R. Leake, M. Gore, and H. Ward), pp. 217–21. RCOG Press, London.

Boronow, R. C., Morrow, C. P., Creasman, W. T., *et al.* (1984). Surgical staging in endometrial cancer: clinical–pathological findings of a prospective study. *Obstetrics and Gynaecology*, 63, 835–42.

Calais, G., Descamps, L., Vitu, L. *et al.* (1990). Lymphadenectomy in the management of endometrial cancer stage I and II. Retrospective study of 155 cases. *Clinical Oncology*, 2, 318–23.

COSA-NZ-UK Endometrial Cancer Study Group (1996). Pelvic lymphadenectomy in high risk endometrial cancer. *International Journal of Gynecological Cancer*, 6, 102–7.

Creasman, W. T., Morrow, C. P., Bundy, B. N. *et al.* (1987). Surgical pathological spread patterns of endometrial cancer. A gynecological oncology group study. *Cancer*, 60, 2035–41.

Gal, D., Rush, S., Lovecchio, J. L. *et al.* (1996). Lymphovascular space involvement—a prognostic indicator in patients with surgical stage I endometrial adenocarcinoma treated with postoperative radiation. *International Journal of Gynecological Cancer*, 6, 135–9.

Grigsby, P. W., Perez, C. A., and Kuten, A. (1992). Prognostic factors for local control and distant metastasis and implications of the new FIGO surgical staging system. *International Journal of Radiation, Oncology, Biology, Physics*, 22, 905–11.

Holmesley, H. D., Kadar, N., Barrett, R. J., and Lentz, S. S. (1992). Selective pelvic and periaortic lymphadenctomy does not increase morbidity in surgical staging of endometrial carcinoma. *American Journal of Obstetrics and Gynecology*, 167, 1225–30.

Kilgore, L. C., Partridge, E. E., Alvarez, R. D. *et al.* (1995). Adenocarcinoma of the endometrium: Survival comparison of patients with and without pelvic node sampling. *Gynecologic Oncology*, 56, 29–33.

Lurain, J. R. (1992). The significance of positive peritoneal cytology in endometrial cancer. *Gynecologic Oncology*, 46, 143–4.

Morrow, C. P., Curtin, J. P., and Townsend, D. E. (ed.) (1993). Uterine sarcomas and related tumours. In *Synopsis of gynecologic oncology*, pp. 189–208. Churchill Livingstone, New York.

Poulsen, H. K., Jacobsen, M., Bertelsen, K. *et al.* (1996). From the Danish Endometrial Cancer Group (DEMCA). Adjuvant radiation therapy is not necessary in the management of endometrial carcinoma stage I, low-risk cases. *International Journal of Gynecological Cancer*, 6, 38–43.

Schink, J. C., Rademaker, A. W., Miller, D. S., and Lurain, J. R. (1991). Tumor size in endometrial cancer. *Cancer*, 67, 2791.

Seoud, C., Johnson, J., and Weed, J. C. (1993). Gynecological tumours in tamoxifen treated women with breast cancer. *Journal of Obstetrics and Gynecology*, 82, 165–9.

Thomas, R. and Blake, P. (1996). Endometrial carcinoma: Adjuvant locoregional therapy. *Clinical Oncology*, 8, 140–5.

Wilson, T. O., Podratz, K. C., Gaffey, T. A. *et al.* (1990). Evaluation of unfavourable histological subtypes in endometrial adenocarcinoma. *American Journal of Obstetrics and Gynecology*, 162, 418–23.

5

Cancer of the vulva and vagina

CANCER OF THE VULVA

Incidence

Vulval cancer is an uncommon gynaecological cancer, mainly affecting elderly women. It accounts for approximately 4 percent of all female genital tumours with an estimated annual incidence of around 3 per 100 000. The life-time risk of developing cancer of the vulva is 0.2 percent. As the majority of women developing vulval cancer are over 65 years of age and as the life expectancy of the female population is increasing, the incidence of vulval cancer is expected to rise.

Aetiology

The aetiology of vulval cancer is not clear. There is often a long history of vulval irritation leading to scratching and further irritation. In some cases viruses may be involved as DNA from human papilloma virus (HPV) types 16 and 18 have been detected in vulval intra-epithelial neoplasia (VIN). The type 2 herpes simplex virus (HSV), may be a co-factor.

Vulval intra-epithelial neoplasia, approximately 40 percent of which occurs in women at or under the age of 40 years, is increasing in incidence. It is similar to cervical intra-epithelial neoplasia, with which it may coexist, but its malignant potential is less than 5 percent. In a few women with un-treated or inadequately treated VIN in whom this progressed to invasive cancer, the latent period was 2–8 years (Jones and Maclean 1986).

Anatomy

The vulva and vagina form the lower part of the reproductive system (Fig. 5.1). The vulva includes the mons pubis, labia majora and minora, clitoris, and vestibule, the latter being the entrance to the vagina into which the urethra opens. They are all covered by squamous epithelium. The mons pubis is a pad of fat covered by hair which is anterior to the pubic symphysis. The labia majora extend from the mons on either side of the vestibule to merge with each other and the perineal skin anterior to the anus at the fourchette. They consist of fat and areolar tissue and have many sebaceous

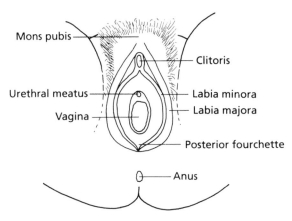

Fig. 5.1 The external anatomy of the vulva and perineum.

glands on their medial surfaces. The labia minora, which are small folds of skin, lie between the labia majora and divide anteriorly to enfold the clitoris, the female equivalent of the penis. The Bartholin's glands (the greater vestibular glands), one on each side, are within the vulva and are apocrine glands that, together with smaller glands in the vaginal mucosa, provide lubrication. They lie in the posterior part of the vestibule and connect to the surface by short ducts.

Lymphatic drainage

The lymphatic drainage is to the inguinal and femoral nodes in the groin. The superficial inguinal nodes are just below the skin along the medial two-thirds of the inguinal ligament and the saphenous vein. The inguinal nodes are the primary nodes which drain the vulva. They drain into the deep femoral nodes located along the femoral artery, vein, and nerve. From there the lymphatic drainage is to the external iliac lymph nodes, the lowest of which, at the entrance of the femoral canal, is known as Cloquet's node and is important as an indicator of the likelihood of metastatic spread to the pelvic nodes. Drainage from midline structures, such as the perineum and clitoris, is to both groins and there is some contralateral drainage from other parts of the vulva.

Spread of disease

Cancer of the vulva involves the labia majora in about two-thirds of patients; and the clitoris, labia minora, posterior fourchette, or perineum in the remainder. Vulval cancer usually spreads slowly and infiltrates local tissues before involving the lymph nodes in the groins. Local spread can extend to involve the vagina, urethra, and anus. Spread to the contralateral groin nodes occurs in 25 percent of cases. Pelvic node involvement is not common and is usually secondary to groin node involvement but rarely there is direct spread to the pelvic nodes via the internal pudendal vessels. Complete obstruction of the lymphatic system can lead to involvement of subcutaneous and dermal lymphatics of the vulva, upper thigh, and lower abdomen. Blood spread to lungs and bone is rare. Unless well managed by a multi-disciplinary team, the terminal stages of this illness, which may be prolonged, can be both painful and unpleasant as a result of infection, ulceration, and incontinence.

Pathology

Vulval intra-epithelial neoplasia (VIN)

The terminology of non-malignant lesions of the vulval skin and mucosa has been defined by the International Society for the Study of Vulvar Disease (1989). This divides the lesions into non-neoplastic disorders and VIN, both squamous and non-squamous (Paget's disease) (Table 5.1). The pathological features of squamous VIN are similar to those of cervical intra-epithelial neoplasia (CIN), with mild to severe dysplasia of the epithelium. VIN is frequently *multi-focal*.

Paget's disease is rare. It presents as a red scaly area. Microscopically, Paget's cells, which are large, pale vacuolated cells with vesicular nuclei, are present in the epidermis. Unlike Paget's disease of the breast, which has a high incidence of underlying adenocarcinoma, no more than one-third of cases of Paget's disease of the vulva is associated with an adenocarcinoma which, if present, is usually of the apocrine glands.

Microinvasive disease

There is now a consensus of opinion that where stromal invasion in vulval cancer is 1 mm or less, there is no associated nodal involvement and inguinal lymphadenectomy is not required. This recognition has led to the inclusion of stage Ia in the new FIGO staging (1996) relating to micro-

Table 5.1 Vulval intra-epithelial neoplasia (VIN): terminology (International Society for the Study of Vulvar Disease 1989)

A. *Squamous VIN*

VIN I   Mild dysplasia

VIN II   Moderate dysplasia

VIN III   Severe dysplasia or carcinoma *in situ*

B. *Non-squamous VIN*

Paget's disease

Table 5.2 Staging of carcinoma of the vulva (FIGO 1996)

Stage	Features
0	Pre-invasive carcinoma (VIN)
I	Tumour confined to vulva or perineum. No lymph node metastases
Ia	Lesions 2 cm or less in size confined to the vulva or perineum with stromal invasion[a] no greater than 1.0 mm
Ib	Lesions 2 cm or less in size confined to the vulva or perineum with stromal invasion[a] greater than 1.0 mm
II	Tumour confined to vulva and/or perineum and more than 2 cm in the greatest dimension. No lymph node metastases
III	Tumour of any size arising on the vulva and/or perineum with adjacent spread to the lower urethra and/or vagina or anus *and/or* Unilateral[b] regional lymph node metastases
IVa	Tumour invading any of the following: upper urethra, bladder mucosa, rectal mucosa, pelvic bone *and/or* Bilateral[b] regional lymph node metastases
IVb	Any distant metastasis including *pelvic* lymph nodes

[a] The depth of invasion is defined as measurement of the tumour from the epithelial stromal junction of the adjacent most superficial dermal papilla to the deepest point of invasion.
[b] Inguinal and femoral lymph nodes.

invasion (Table 5.2). Involvement of the superficial and deep inguinal nodes can occur in all cases with more than 1 mm stromal invasion.

Invasive disease

The majority (85 percent), of vulval cancers are squamous in type. Less than 5 percent are melanomas and the remainder are carcinomas of Bartholin's gland, other adenocarcinomas, basal cell carcinomas, or the very rare verrucous carcinomas, rhabdomyosarcomas, and leiomyosarcomas.

Symptoms and signs

Vulval intra-epithelial neoplasia (VIN)

This often presents as pruritis vulvae but 20–45 percent of cases are asymptomatic and are most frequently found after previous treatment of CIN or cancer of the cervix or anus. The lesions are often raised and vary in colour from white due to hyperkeritinization, red due to immaturity of the epithelium, to brown due to increased deposition of melanin in the epithelial cells (Soutter 1993). The full extent of the lesion becomes apparent, when examined colposcopically, after the application of 5 percent acetic acid. The VIN turns white but the lesions are more difficult to examine than in CIN, and all abnormal areas should be biopsied to confirm the diagnosis.

Invasive disease

Most patients with cancer of the vulva (70 percent) complain of irritation or pruritis and 57 percent report a vulval mass or ulcer. Bleeding occurs in 28 percent and discharge in 23 percent (Monaghan 1985). Frequently, it is not until a mass is present that advice is sought and delays of several months are not uncommon between the onset of symptoms and referral to a gynaecologist. This is not only due to the reluctance of an elderly woman to seek advice but is also due to the initial medical investigation failing to recognize the condition resulting in inappropriate treatment. Occasionally, enlarged inguinal nodes are the first abnormality noticed by the patient.

Investigations

All patients with VIN must be examined for evidence of *in situ* and invasive cancer elsewhere in the genital tract as 'field' changes may be present. Clinical evaluation for invasive disease of the vulva, includes cervical cytology and, if necessary, colposcopy and biopsy of the cervix in addition to examination of the vulva and vagina. The inguinal nodes should be palpated and, if enlarged, a fine needle aspirate performed, for cytological examination, to distinguish between infection and malignancy.

Examination under anaesthesia and a *full thickness* biopsy of the lesion are the most important investigations both to confirm the diagnosis and to determine the extent of the lesion, noting its size and involvement of other structures such as the urethra or anus.

Other investigations include full blood count, serum biochemistry, and chest X-ray. In advanced disease imaging of the pelvis and abdomen by computerized tomography (CT) or magnetic resonance imaging (MRI) scanning should be carried out to identify the full extent of disease.

Clinical staging

The FIGO classification for cancer of the vulva is shown on Table 5.2. This is a *surgical* staging as pathological assessment is the only accurate method of determining lymph node involvement. Clinical assessment of lymph node status, which is an important prognostic indicator, is inaccurate. The overall incidence of lymph node metastases in the groin, in the absence of clinical findings, is around 30 percent.

Prognostic factors

The most important prognostic factors are FIGO stage and the presence of *clinically* involved inguinal lymph nodes. The effect of stage and nodal involvement on survival is shown in Tables 5.3 and 5.4. As expected, increasing stage is indicative of a poorer prognosis and the effect of inguino-femoral node involvement on survival depends both on the number of involved nodes and whether they are unilateral or bilateral. In the Gynecologic Oncology Group (GOG) series shown in Table 5.4 it can be seen that there were no survivors in this study when more than 6 nodes were involved with tumour (Holmesley *et al.* 1991). Pelvic node involvement, stage IVb, indicates that the disease has spread beyond the regional nodes, and this is associated with a very poor prognosis.

The other important prognostic features that are indicative of the likelihood of lymph node involvement are tumour size, tumour location, with midline tumours having a worse prognosis than laterally situated

Table 5.3 Results, according to stage, of treatment of squamous carcinoma of the vulva (modified from FIGO 1988)

Stage	No. of patients (%)	5-year survival (%)
I	30.5	69
II	32	49
III	28.5	32
IV	7	13

Table 5.4 Influence of groin node status on survival in squamous carcinoma of the vulva (377 patients) (GOG. 1991)

Groin node status	5-year survival (%)
Negative	92
Positive	
Ipsilateral	75
Bilateral	30
Contralateral	27
>2 nodes	25
>6 nodes	0

Table 5.5 Risk groups for vulval carcinoma

| Risk group | Surgical–pathological findings | | Survival at 5 years (%) |
	Tumour diameter	Groin node status	
Minimal	< or equal to 2 cm	Negative	98
Low	2.1–8 cm	Negative	87
	< or equal to 2 cm	Positive: 1	
Intermediate	>8 cm	Negative	75
	2.1–8 cm	Positive: 1 or 2	
High	>8 cm	Positive:2	29
	Any size	Positive: 3 or more ipsilateral	
	Any size	Bilateral	

Modified from Holmesley *et al.* (1991). A GOG study.

tumours on account of their increased tendency to metastasize to both groins, age and performance status. The effect of increasing tumour size on survival is shown in Table 5.5 where, in the GOG study (Holmesley *et al.* 1991), tumour size and nodal status have been used to divide risk groups into minimal, low, intermediate, and high.

The most significant *pathological* features are the presence and number of involved inguinal nodes and the width of the tumour-free margin in the vulva. If the latter is less than 8 mm there is a serious risk of local tumour recurrence following surgery.

The other pathological variables of prognostic significance indicate the likelihood of lymphatic involvement. They are high grade of tumour, depth of tumour greater than 1 mm, presence of lympho-vascular space invasion, perineural invasion, and tumour border pattern (infiltrating vs pushing) (Heaps *et al.* 1990; Hopkins *et al.* 1991). Tumours of high grade are more likely to invade deeply. Morrow *et al.* (1993) collated data from five reports and found no incidence of groin node metastases in clinical stage I squamous carcinoma of the vulva in lesions invading 1 mm or less, but this rose to 8 percent for a depth of 1–2 mm, 11 percent for 2–3 mm, and over 25 percent for lesions of greater than 3 mm depth.

Spread to the pelvic nodes is rare if the ipsilateral inguinal nodes are clear. If the inguinal nodes are involved the overall risk of pelvic node involvement is approximately 20 percent. The risk is low in histologically positive inguinal nodes which appear to be clinically free of tumour. However, the risk increases when the nodes are *clinically* involved, or when there is metastasis to three or more ipsilateral, inguinal nodes, or bilateral involvement.

Treatment

Surgery

Vulval intraepithelial neoplasia (VIN)

The treatment for this disease is difficult because of its multi-focal nature. Asymptomatic patients, particularly under the age of 50 years, are probably best observed regularly and biopsies repeated if there are any suspicious changes (Soutter 1993).

The main treatment is surgery. The advantage of surgery is that one can ensure that the lesion has been completely removed and that an early malignancy has not been missed. For small unifocal lesions a wide local excision of the epidermis with a good margin suffices. If the disease is extensive or multi-focal more extensive surgery with plastic surgery may be required.

Vaporization of VIN, with the carbon dioxide laser, has been used as an alternative treatment to surgery but the depth of tissue that needs to be treated can vary from 1 mm in non-hairy areas to 3 mm where hair is present, as hair follicles may be involved up to 2.6 mm below the skin surface (Shatz *et al.* 1989). Vaporization can give a good cosmetic result but only if the lesion is superficial and is not involving a large area. Repeat treatments may be necessary.

Invasive disease

The treatment of choice for cancer of the vulva is surgery. Until recently the standard surgical treatment has been radical vulvectomy which involves removing the vulva with wide margins of skin and subcutaneous tissue and carrying out a bilateral groin node dissection of both the superficial and deep nodes. This operation was originally carried out by Taussig (1949) and was modified by Way in 1960. The disadvantage of this operation was that large areas of normal skin were removed from the groins and primary wound closure was seldom achieved. Monaghan (1986) modified the incision to allow primary healing after radical vulvectomy and Hacker *et al.* (1981) advocated the use of separate groin incisions (Fig. 5.2).

There is a move to more conservative surgical treatment of the vulva for early stage disease. A proposed technique is 'radical' local excision, in order to reduce the side-effects of the surgery with regard to both body image and sexuality, and to improve recovery. The benefits of such an approach are less in anterior and clitoral lesions.

Lymphadenectomy, confined to the ipsilateral inguinal and femoral nodes, is advocated for small lesions with no clinical suspicion of nodal involvement, although if pathological positive nodes are found the contra-lateral nodes will need to be excised at a later date. Patients with vulval lesions no larger than 2 cm, with a depth of less than 1 mm, and no lympho-

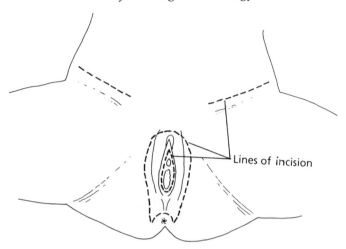

Lines of incision

Fig. 5.2 Lines of excision for a radical vulvectomy.

vascular space involvement, are unlikely to have nodal involvement and do not require lymphadenectomy.

If the inguinal nodes are involved, post-operative radiotherapy to the groins and pelvis has been shown to be superior to pelvic lymphadenectomy, in terms of improved 2-year survival rates and fewer groin recurrences (Holmesley *et al.* 1986).

Post-operative complications, which include leg oedema in about 30 percent of patients and numbness over the anterior thigh from the division of branches of the femoral nerve, as well as delayed wound healing, are discussed in Chapter 8.

Radiotherapy

Surgery is the mainstay of treatment for vulval carcinoma but, in the presence of advanced disease with bowel or bladder involvement, surgery can result in poor function and cosmesis. This has led to a renewed interest in the use of the non-surgical modalities of radiotherapy and chemotherapy (Harrington and Lambert 1994).

External beam radiotherapy is poorly tolerated by the thin epithelium of the vulva, leading to acute moist desquamation and severe late normal tissue damage in the form of vulval fibrosis, atrophy and necrosis, urethral stenosis, and fistula formation. However, these complications can be avoided by using smaller daily doses per fraction (e.g. 1.6–1.8 Gy), and by limiting the overall total dose. Thomas *et al.* (1989, 1991) advise that the upper limit for total dose, at this fractionation, should be 55 Gy *pre-operatively*, which is a lower than radical dose, in order not to interfere with wound healing after surgery; 45–50 Gy *post-operatively* as adjuvant treatment; 65 Gy *as radical treatment.* Doses of over 70 Gy to the vulva are associated with necrosis.

However, the optimal fractionation regimen has not yet been determined. Thomas *et al.* (1989) found that prolonged treatment breaks (10–34 days, median 19 days) were necessary in 60 percent of 27 patients treated with radiotherapy and concomitant chemotherapy using 5-fluorouracil and mitomycin C. Daily fractions of 1.6–1.8 Gy were given to the vulva, to a total dose of 40–64 Gy and 36–59 Gy to the inguinal nodes. This delay would only have been due in part to the chemotherapy.

An alternative method is to give twice-daily fractionation using 1.5 Gy per fraction with a 6-hour gap, giving 30 fractions in 3 weeks, to a total dose of 45 Gy to the vulva. In those patients not proceeding to surgery the treatment is continued to 64.5 Gy, usually to a smaller volume, following a planned 2-week gap to allow skin healing and shrinkage of the tumour (Soutter *et al.* 1995).

It is important when treating the vulva with radiation to limit the size of the treatment field to reduce long-term morbidity. This is achieved by selecting the most appropriate techniques, such as direct perineal electron portals or interstitial radiotherapy for localized lesions. When the whole vulva needs to be treated, opposed anterior and posterior fields are used. Sometimes, interstitial treatment is given following external radiotherapy but the total dose remains the same.

Post-operative radiotherapy

Up to one-third of patients with advanced operable disease recur after radical surgery and in almost all of these patients this will occur initially in loco-regional sites.

The criteria for post-operative radiotherapy to the nodes, both inguinal and pelvic, have been specified as the presence of a single *clinically* involved inguinal node or two or more *histologically* involved nodes or *extracapsular spread* (Thomas *et al.* 1991). A typical radiation dose for post-operative radiotherapy to the groins and pelvic nodes is 45–50 Gy at 1.8–2.0 Gy per fraction.

A surgical disease-free margin of 1 cm for the vulval carcinoma is consistent with a high degree of local control but a margin of less than 8 mm is associated with a 50 percent chance of recurrence (Heaps *et al.* 1990). The choice of treatment is close observation, further surgery, or radiotherapy. The radiotherapy treatment field can be small as it is confined to the site of the tumour. The recommended dose, as stated earlier, is 45–50 Gy.

Radiotherapy as an alternative to surgery for occult nodal disease

Occult nodal metastases are present in 20–25 percent of women with impalpable nodes. The question has been raised whether radiotherapy could be used in place of inguinal lymphadenectomy to reduce the morbidity of surgery. However, a GOG study which randomized patients, with no suspicious inguinal nodes, to receive node dissection or inguino-femoral node irradiation was terminated prematurely when an interim analysis showed a significant advantage for the surgical arm (Stehman *et al.* 1992). Although there are criticisms of this study, radiotherapy cannot be recommended as an alternative to surgery for occult nodal disease at the present time.

Pre-operative radiotherapy

Pre-operative radiotherapy and/or chemotherapy has been used to try to reduce advanced tumours to enable subsequent surgery to be 'viscera-preserving'. The largest study by Boronow *et al.* (1987), showed benefit for pre-operative radiotherapy in 48 women, 11 of whom had recurrent disease with a projected 5-year survival of 76 percent for the primary cases and 63 percent for the recurrent cases. Only 2 patients subsequently required an exenterative procedure or stoma formation. The value of pre-operative radiotherapy for clinically involved nodes has also been demonstrated.

More recently, chemoradiotherapy has been assessed for the treatment of advanced cancer of the vulva with the chemotherapy being used as a radio-sensitizer rather than as a cytotoxic agent. Results have been mixed and most of the studies have been very small. In a larger study, results were obtained in 20 patients by Koh *et al.* (1993). Their regimen was to treat bulk disease to a maximum of 70 Gy and areas at risk of microscopic spread to 54 Gy. Chemotherapy was 5-fluorouracil (5FU) and cisplatin. At sphincter-preserving surgery the response rate was found to be 90 percent with 10 complete pathological responses and 8 partial responses. It would appear that radiotherapy or chemoradiotherapy has a role in 'down-staging' advanced tumours prior to surgery but more studies are needed to define the best pre-operative radiotherapy regimen for vulval carcinoma.

Primary radical non-surgical treatment

Radical radiotherapy as the main treatment for vulval cancer has been little used but several small studies using chemoradiotherapy, as given above, have shown this to be an effective treatment with salvage surgery reserved for local failures. Similar treatment for cancer of the anus has been highly successful and has saved patients from stoma formation. In advanced vulval cancer, radiotherapy, alone or with chemotherapy, should be considered where surgical treatment would result in considerable morbidity with loss of organs such as the bladder or rectum.

Chemotherapy

Chemotherapy has not had a large role to play in the management of vulval carcinoma probably because of the advanced age of the patients and the frequency of concurrent medical conditions. Single agents that have been shown to have activity include cisplatin, doxorubicin, bleomycin, and methotrexate. Cisplatin, 5FU, and bleomycin have all been used with radio-therapy as radiosensitizers but no randomized studies have been carried out to show whether chemoradiotherapy is superior to radiotherapy alone.

Chemotherapy has also been studied in the neoadjuvant setting by the EORTC Gynecological Cancer Co-operative Group (Durrant *et al.* 1990) to give a low intensity, continuous regimen for elderly women with advanced disease. The drugs used were, bleomycin, methotrexate, and carmustine (CCNU). One-third of the 31 patients evaluated failed to complete the treatment, confirming the toxicity of this treatment modality in elderly and unfit women.

Summary

1. Radical surgery, by wide excision or vulvectomy and bilateral inguino-femoral lymphadenectomy, is the main treatment for cancer of the vulva. Lesser vulval surgery is being considered for early stage disease but, except for lesions of 1 mm depth or less, ipsilateral or bilateral inguino-femoral lymphadenectomy is necessary because of the high risk of nodal involvement.

2. Radiotherapy is given post-operatively to the pelvic nodes and inguinal areas in the presence of nodal metastases. It also has a role in the prevention of local recurrence in the vulva and pre-operatively to reduce tumour size in patients with advanced disease.

3. Chemotherapy has been little used because of the age and medical condition of the majority of women who develop this disease. Its main role is as concomitant treatment with radiotherapy but whether this is better than radiotherapy alone has not been established.

Results

Published 5-year survival rates for invasive cancer vary widely due to the low incidence of this tumour and the advanced age of the majority of patients. The FIGO results are shown in Table 5.3. With negative groin nodes the 5-year survival rates range from 69 percent to 100 percent, but when more than two groin nodes are positive or contralateral nodes are involved the survival rates are poor (Table 5.4). With pelvic node involvement the 5-year survival drops to 20 percent.

Conclusions

Epithelial carcinoma of the vulva is an uncommon tumour which mainly affects elderly women. Delays in patients seeking advice and in making the diagnosis result in tumours being frequently advanced at the time treatment is commenced. The incidence of vulval intra-epithelial neoplasia is increasing, especially in young women and presents a problem in treatment because of its multi-focal nature and the need to avoid mutilating therapy. Treatment for both pre-invasive and invasive disease is surgical but radiotherapy and chemoradiotherapy have an increasing role in the management of advanced vulval cancer.

Uncommon tumours of the vulva

Malignant melanoma (of the vulva and vagina)

Malignant melanoma of the vulva and vagina accounts for 3 percent of the total incidence of melanomas and comprise less than 5 percent of vulvo-vaginal malignancies. More than 90 percent of the melanomas occurs in the vulva, where it is the second most common vulval tumour. The lesions vary from black to completely amelanotic.

The prognosis is related to the depth of the tumour and is good for a depth of less than 0.76 mm. Breslow's classification of melanoma is divided into five levels and measures the distance from the surface epithelium to the point of deepest penetration (Table 5.6) (Breslow 1970). Invasion occurs in an *outward direction as well as a downward direction* so a wide excision is required. This is usually radical vulvectomy, without lymphadenectomy unless the nodes are involved. Other forms of therapy, such as radiotherapy, chemotherapy, or immunotherapy have had very little impact on this disease.

Five-year survival for patients without nodal involvement is around 56 percent falling to 14 percent when metastatic spread to the nodes has occurred (Morrow and DiSaia 1976). Melanoma of the vagina has a particularly bad prognosis with a 5-year survival of around 10 percent.

Basal cell carcinoma

Basal cell carcinomas may occur in the skin at any site including the vulva. They are only locally invasive and are treated by local excision with excellent results.

Table 5.6 Classification of melanoma (Breslow 1970)

Level	Thickness of lesion (mm)
1	<0.76
2	0.76–1.5
3	1.51–3.0
4	>3.0–4.0
5	>4.0

Bartholin's gland carcinoma

These tumours are usually adenocarcinomas, although rarely they may have adenosquamous, or pure squamous pathology. They are usually diagnosed late when spread to the groin and pelvic nodes has already occurred. Treatment is radical vulvectomy and bilateral inguino-femoral lymph-adenectomy.

Adenoid cystic tumours of Bartholin's gland can also occur. They behave in the same way as adenoid cystic tumours found in salivary glands, that is, they spread by local invasion and along neural sheaths, making complete excision difficult. Treatment is by radical surgery but radiotherapy is useful in recurrent disease.

Verrucous carcinoma of the vulva

Verrucous carcinoma of the vulva is a very rare variant of an epithelial tumour which, with its papillary growth, resembles condyloma acuminata. Histologically, it is difficult to distinguish this tumour from a benign lesion unless a deep biopsy is taken. Verrucous carcinomas are locally invasive but seldom metastasize to the inguinal nodes. The usual treatment is surgery, either wide excision for small lesions or vulvectomy, but there is no indication to remove the inguinal nodes. Radiotherapy was considered to be contra-indicated in verrucous carcinomas as it was thought to result in dedifferentiation of the tumour, but this is no longer considered to be true.

Sarcomas

These rare tumours of the vulva include leiomyosarcomas, which tend to grow slowly and metastasize late, and rhabdomyosarcomas, which are rapidly growing aggressive tumours. A radical vulvectomy and groin node dissection is the usual treatment, but local recurrence and blood-borne metastases are common. The prognosis is very poor.

CANCER OF THE VAGINA

Incidence

Cancer of the vagina is a rare tumour which mainly affects elderly women. It comprises only 1–2 percent of all gynaecological malignancies, the incidence being less than 1 per 100 000 women and the lifetime risk less than 0.1 percent. The upper third of the vagina is the most common site for the cancer to occur, 25–30 percent arise in the lower third while the middle third is the least common site of origin. Most vaginal cancers are advanced at the time of diagnosis.

Cancer found in the vagina is usually as a result of direct spread from cervical or vulval cancer, or it is metastatic (e.g. from the endometrium, bladder, or large bowel). Therefore, before making a diagnosis of primary vaginal cancer the following criteria must be met: the primary site of growth must be in the vagina, the cervix and vulva must not be involved, and there must be no evidence that the vaginal tumour is metastatic from a primary elsewhere.

Vaginal intra-epithelial neoplasia (VAIN), is now being seen more frequently. It is more common following hysterectomy and is usually multi-focal and, although some lesions may be extensions of cervical intra-epithelial neoplasia (CIN), it also occurs *de novo*. Like CIN it can progress to invasive cancer.

Aetiology

The aetiology of vaginal cancer is obscure. A few cases may be caused by chronic irritation from a procidentia, pessary, or frequent vaginal douching. Previous radiotherapy for cervical cancer in young women has also been suggested as a cause of cancer of the vagina, but this is an uncommon event. In some women, there appears to be a 'field' effect, in that multi-centric cancers can arise affecting cervix, vagina, vulva and, occasionally, the anus as well. As with cancer of the cervix, human papilloma virus (HPV) has been suggested as an aetiological agent.

The use of diethylstilboestrol in pregnancy, thus exposing the fetus to excess oestrogens, was thought to be responsible for many cases of clear cell adenocarcinoma of the vagina. However, although oestrogen exposure causes vaginal adenosis (the abnormal presence of glandular tissue in the squamous epithelium), the risk of vaginal cancer is now considered to be relatively low, between 0.1 and 1.0 per 1000 exposed fetuses. Nevertheless, the incidence of CIN is increased in women who were exposed to intra-uterine diethylstilboestrol.

Anatomy

Embryologically, the upper two-thirds of the vagina develops separately from the lower third, the upper part growing down from the Mullerian ducts and the lower third developing upwards from the cloaca, thus sharing its blood and lymphatic system with that of the vulva. It is lined throughout by stratified squamous epithelium. The cervix protrudes into the vaginal vault superiorly and the vagina meets the vulva at the vestibule inferiorly (Fig. 5.3). Anteriorly, the vagina is related to the bladder and urethra, and posteriorly, where it is covered by the peritoneum, it is related to loops of

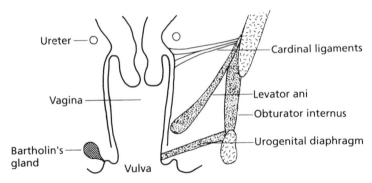

Fig. 5.3 Coronal section of the vagina and vulva showing the relationship of the vagina to the muscles of the pelvic floor and to Bartholin's gland.

bowel in the pouch of Douglas. Below the peritoneal cavity it is in close proximity to the anterior wall of the rectum and is separated from the anus by the perineal body. The ureters, close to the cervix, pass near to each side of the vaginal vault. The vagina is supported laterally by the lower part of the cardinal ligaments until it reaches the pelvic floor where it is surrounded by the medial part of the levator ani muscles.

Lymphatic drainage

The lymphatic drainage of the upper two-thirds of the vagina is to the pelvic nodes, similar to the lymphatic drainage of the cervix (Fig. 3.5, p. 50). The drainage of the lower third is similar to that of the vulva, draining first into the inguinal and femoral nodes and thence into the pelvic nodes, reflecting the different embryological origin of the upper and lower vagina.

Spread of disease

Vaginal cancer spreads by local invasion to the rest of the vagina, vulva, paravaginal tissues, and parametria. Lymphatic spread to the pelvic nodes from the upper two-thirds of the vagina occurs in less than 10% of patients with tumours limited to the vaginal mucosa (stage I) but rises to approximately 25% if the parametria are involved (stage II). Inguinal node involvement occurs in approximately one-third of cancers originating in the lower third of the vagina. Haematogenous spread is unusual and occurs late.

Pathology

Vaginal intra-epithelial neoplasia (VAIN) is classified in a similar manner to cervical intra-epithelial neoplasia (CIN), relating grade to loss of stratification and nuclear atypia. It must be considered to have malignant potential. VAIN usually occurs in the upper posterior vagina but about 25–30 percent of cases are confined to the lower vagina, usually the anterior wall.

More than 90 percent of primary invasive tumours of the vagina are squamous in type, 4–5 percent are adenocarcinomas and rarely malignant melanomas and sarcomas occur.

Symptoms and signs

Vaginal intra-epithelial neoplasia (VAIN)

The diagnosis of VAIN is usually made on cytological or colposcopic examination. A vaginal smear showing dyskariotic cells needs assessment by colposcopy to find the origin of these cells and to take a biopsy. In those patients who have had a hysterectomy VAIN can occur around the suture line or in the angles of the vault, resulting in difficulties in assessment and biopsy. It is important to rule out invasive disease behind the suture line. When assessing patients with abnormal cytology the complete vagina should be inspected as the blades of a bivalve speculum can obscure VAIN.

Invasive disease

Symptoms

As a result of the increased use of cytology for screening, some women are detected before they develop symptoms. The majority, however, present at an advanced stage with postmenopausal bleeding as the commonest symptom. Vaginal discharge, urinary symptoms, and pelvic pain are less common and are suggestive of advanced disease.

Investigations

The most important investigation is examination under anaesthesia. This should include careful inspection of the whole vagina and cervix, a combined vaginal and rectal examination to detect extra-vaginal spread and cystoscopy. Biopsies are taken of abnormal lesions and must be full-thickness for accurate histological diagnosis.

Other investigations include blood indices, renal and liver function tests, and radiological assessment of the renal tract. In more advanced cases CT or MRI scanning of the abdomen and pelvis to assess nodal involvement and the extent of the disease is necessary. Ultrasound can also help to define the size and extent of the primary particularly if this is carried out using a transrectal or transvaginal probe.

Table 5.7 Modified FIGO staging of vaginal carcinoma

Stage	Features
0	Pre-invasive carcinoma (VAIN)
I	Carcinoma limited to vaginal mucosa
IIa	Involvement of subvaginal tissues: not extending to parametrium
IIb	Parametrial involvement not extending to pelvic side wall
III	Carcinoma extends to pelvic side wall
IVa	Involvement of mucosa of bladder or rectum
IVb	Spread beyond the pelvis

Staging

The FIGO staging for vaginal cancer is shown on Table 5.7. Staging for cancer of the vagina is based on *clinical* findings. One-third of women will be stage I at presentation, one-third stage II, and the remainder either stage III or IV.

Prognostic factors

Stage is the most important prognostic sign, as it relates to the spread of disease through the vaginal mucosa and involvement of other local tissues. High grade of tumour, which tends to be associated with both large tumours and increased depth of penetration, also has a poor prognosis, as does the presence of lymph node involvement.

Treatment

Vaginal intra-epithelial neoplasia (VAIN)

The main treatments for vaginal intra-epithelial neoplasia are local ablation, surgery, and radiotherapy. Local application of 5-fluorouracil is no longer recommended. Local ablation with the carbon dioxide laser is used for small lesions where there is no suspicion of invasion. Local excision is sufficient for small single lesions, otherwise partial or total colpectomy (vaginectomy) is necessary. The latter may require the formation of a neo-vagina to enable sexual function to be preserved but does not preclude vaginal cancer subsequently developing in the neo-vagina. Intracavitary radiotherapy is an option for lesions in the vaginal vault following a hysterectomy, but this will have the disadvantage of causing vaginal stenosis and, if the woman is premenopausal, ovarian failure.

Invasive disease

The treatment of vaginal cancer is by radiotherapy, although in a few cases surgery is preferred. As most cases of vaginal cancer present late in an elderly population radical treatment is not always possible.

Surgery

Local excision can be carried out for small stage I lesions if an adequate margin of the tumour can be obtained. For cancer in the uppermost part of the vagina, radical hysterectomy and pelvic lymphadenectomy is needed, as for cancer of the cervix, as well as partial or complete vaginectomy and the formation of a neo-vagina. Following surgery, there can be problems with urinary continence. Vaginal reconstruction should be offered but is not always successful, sometimes leading to discharge, stenosis, and prolapse.

If the vaginal cancer is stage IV, or recurs locally after previous radiotherapy, exenteration may, occasionally, be feasible.

Radiotherapy

Most patients with vaginal carcinoma are treated with radiotherapy which is given either as a combination of external radiation and brachytherapy or by brachytherapy alone. Radiotherapy is particularly useful for stage I lesions which would otherwise require extensive surgery.

Combined therapy: external radiotherapy and brachytherapy

Tumours of the upper two-thirds of the vagina are treated in an identical fashion to cancer of the cervix, by external radiotherapy to the pelvis to include the parametria and the pelvic nodes. The lower end of the field must cover the lesion in the vagina plus a 2 cm margin. If the lesion extends into the lower third of the vagina the inguino-femoral nodes must also be included in the treatment volume. A total dose of 45–50 Gy in 25–28 fractions in 5–6 weeks, is given to the pelvis. External radiotherapy is followed by intracavitary therapy, using an intrauterine tube and ovoids, for lesions limited to the vaginal vault. For lesions below the vault, the treatment boost is with an interstitial implant or by intracavitary treatment using a vaginal obturator. Interstitial brachytherapy has been found to be more effective than intracavitary treatment for lesions below the vault (Stock *et al.* 1992). However, if the tumour has been found to have completely regressed following external irradiation, brachytherapy, using a vaginal obturator, will give a sufficient dose to the vaginal mucosa. The total dose, to include low dose rate brachytherapy, is 70–75 Gy to the vaginal mucosa, or its equivalent using a high dose rate system.

Brachytherapy, interstitial, as sole treatment

In the middle and lower third of the vagina, early tumours (stage I and IIa) that are less than 2–3 cm in diameter are ideally treated with an interstitial implant alone, using an after-loading technique with iridium-192 wires. The geometry of the implant is improved by the use of a plastic template to hold rigidly the steel tubes that carry the iridium wires (Fig. 5.4). In the Hammersmith Hospital template, based on the Syed–Neblett applicator, iridium-192 is after-loaded into three concentric rings of stainless steel guide needles (Branson *et al.* 1985). The two outer rings of needles are inserted under general anaesthesia, through the perineum, into the paravaginal space. The inner ring is located in grooves on the vaginal obturator. A total dose of 70–80 Gy at a rate of 10 Gy per day, is given in 2 insertions 2 weeks apart, unless the lesion is small when 60 Gy is given in 1 insertion over 6 days.

External radiotherapy as sole treatment

Stage IVa tumours are treated by external radiotherapy alone as the treatment is given with palliative intent.

Complications

Radiotherapy leads to vaginal stenosis in up to one-third of patients, particularly when advanced tumours are treated, but this complication can

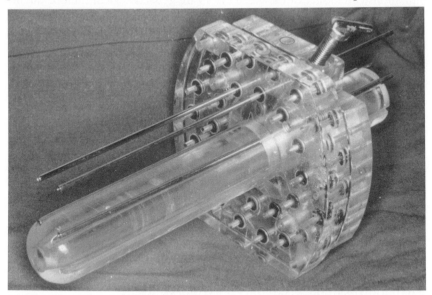

Fig. 5.4 The perspex template for holding parallel, after-loading tubes for use with iridium-192 wire. The template is stitched to the perineum with the central obturator in the vagina. The after-loading tubes are introduced with the aid of a trochar.

be reduced by the use of vaginal douches during treatment and vaginal dilators following treatment. Delayed healing of the vaginal mucosa usually responds to conservative treatment.

Chemotherapy

The use of cytotoxic drugs in vaginal carcinoma is extremely limited. However, as neoadjuvant or concomitant treatment, or for palliating recurrent disease in younger women the same drugs can be used as for cancer of the cervix.

Results

Owing to the rarity of this disease there is a wide range of reported results. One report (Kuçera and Vavra 1991) looked at the outcome in 434 patients with vaginal cancer. Their findings showed that 77 percent of patients with stage I disease were alive at 5 years compared to 45 percent with stage II, 31 percent with stage III, and 18 percent with stage IV disease.

Conclusions

Squamous carcinoma of the vagina is a rare gynaecological tumour mainly affecting elderly women. It is usually already advanced at diagnosis. VAIN is becoming more frequent in younger women, particularly in association with CIN. While surgery is the main treatment for VAIN, invasive cancer is usually treated with radiotherapy.

Other vaginal tumours

Clear cell adenocarcinomas

These tumours occur either at around 20 years of age or in women aged 60 years or over. The histology of these rare tumours, which are occasionally associated with intrauterine exposure to stilboestrol, is characterized by vacuolated or clear areas in the cytoplasm and a hobnail appearance of the nuclei of the cells lining the glands. Most are situated in the upper vagina and metastasis to pelvic lymph nodes can occur. The treatment is radical surgery or radical radiotherapy in a similar fashion to cervical cancer. The prognosis is similar to that of cervical cancer.

Rhabdomyosarcoma (sarcoma botyroides)

The majority of these tumours (90 percent), occur in girls under the age of 5 years. Macroscopically, a grape-like mass protrudes from the vagina. The presenting symptom is vaginal bleeding.

Rhabdomyosarcoma is sensitive to chemotherapy which produces both complete and partial responses. Treatment needs to be carried out in a specialist centre as those children with incomplete responses are subsequently treated with local surgery. Occasionally, exenteration is required for resistant disease. Radiotherapy is restricted to patients with unresectable tumour in view of the deleterious effects on bone growth. An overall survival rate of over 80 percent is achieved.

Malignant melanoma

Malignant melanoma of the vagina is a very rare tumour. It has been discussed earlier in this chapter (p. 110), together with malignant melanoma of the vulva.

References

Cancer of the vulva

Breslow, A. (1970). Thickness, cross-sectional areas, and depth of invasion in the prognosis of cutaneous melanoma. *Annals of Surgery*, **172**, 902–8.

Boronow, R. C., Hickman, B. T., Reagan, M. T. *et al.* (1987). Combined therapy as an alternative to exenteration for locally advanced vulvovaginal cancer. *American Journal of Clinical Oncology*, **10**, 171–81.

Durrant, K. R., Mangionin, C., Lacave, A. J. *et al.* (1990). Bleomycin, methotrexate, and CCNU in advanced inoperable squamous cell carcinoma of the vulva: a Phase II study of the EORTC Gynecological Cancer Co-operative Group (GCCG). *Gynecologic Oncology*, **37**, 359–62.

Hacker, N. F., Leuchter, R. S., Berek, J. S. *et al.* (1981). Radical vulvectomy and bilateral inguinal lymphadenectomy through separate groin incisions. *Obstetrics and Gynecology*, **58**, 574–9.

Harrington, K. J. and Lambert, H. E. (1994). Current issues in the non-surgical management of primary vulvar squamous cell carcinoma. *Clinical Oncology*, **6**, 331–6.

Heaps, J. M., Fu, Y. S., Montz, F. J. *et al.* (1990). Surgical-pathological variables predictive of local recurrence in squamous carcinoma of the vulva. *Gynecologic Oncology*, **38**, 309–14.

Holmesley, H. D., Bundy, B. N., Sedlis, A., and Adcock, L. (1986). Radiation therapy versus pelvic node resection for carcinoma of the vulva with positive groin nodes. *Obstetrics and Gynecology*, **68**, 733–40.

Holmesley, H. D., Bundy, B. N., Sedlis, A. *et al.* (1991). Assessment of current International Federation of Gynecology and Obstetrics staging of vulvar carcinoma relative to prognostic factors for survival: a Gynecologic Oncology Group Study. *American Journal of Obstetrics and Gynecology*, **164**, 997–1004.

Hopkins, M. P., Reid, G. C., Vettrano, I. *et al.* (1991). Squamous cell carcinoma of the vulva: prognostic factors influencing survival. *Gynecologic Oncology*, **43**, 113–17.

International Society for the Study of Vulvar Disease (1989). New nomenclature for vulvar disease. Report of the committee on terminology. *American Journal of Obstetrics and Gynecology*, 73, 769.

Jones, R. W. and McLean, M. R. (1986). Carcinoma in situ of the vulva: a review of 31 treated and five untreated cases. *Obstetrics and Gynecology*, 68, 499–503.

Koh, W. J., Wallace, H. J., Greer, B. E. *et al.* (1993). Combined radiotherapy and chemotherapy in the management of local-regionally advanced vulvar cancer. *International Journal of Radiation, Oncology, Biology, Physics*, 26, 809–16.

Monaghan, J. M. (1985). Management of vulvar carcinoma. In *Clinical gynaecological oncology* (ed. J. H. Shepherd and J. M. Monaghan), pp. 133–53. Blackwell, London.

Monaghan, J. M. (1986). Radical surgery for carcinoma of the vulva. In *Bonney's gynaecological surgery* (3rd edn.) (ed. J. M. Monaghan), pp. 121–8. Ballière Tindall, Eastbourne.

Morrow, C. P. and DiSaia, P. J. (1976). Malignant melanoma of the female genitalia: a clinical analysis. *Obstetrics Gynecologic Survey*, 31, 233–71.

Morrow, C. P., Curtin, J. P., and Townsend, D. E. (ed.) (1993). Tumours of the vulva. In *Synopsis of gynecologic oncology* (4th edn.), pp. 65–92.

Shatz, P., Bergeron, C., Wilkinson, E. J. *et al.* (1989). Vulvar intraepithelial neoplasia and skin appendage involvement. *Obstetrics and Gynecology*, 74, 769–74.

Soutter, P. (1993). *Colposcopy of the vulva in practical colposcopy*, pp. 161–86. Oxford University Press.

Soutter, W. P., Lambert, H. E., and McIndoe, G. A. J. (1995). Carcinoma of the vulva and its putative precursors. In *Oxford textbook of oncology* (ed. S. T. Peckham, B. Pindeo, and U. Veronesi), pp. 1383–94. Oxford University Press.

Stehman, F. B., Bundy, B. N., Thomas, G. *et al.* (1992). Groin dissection versus groin radiation in carcinoma of the vulva. A Gynecologic Oncology Group Study. *International Journal of Radiation, Oncology, Biology, Physics*, 24, 389–96.

Taussig, F. J. (1949). Cancer of the vulva: An analysis of 155 cases (1991–1940). *American Journal of Obstetrics and Gynecology*, 40, 764–79.

Thomas, G., Dembo, A., DePetrillo, A. *et al.* (1989). Concurrent radiation and chemotherapy in vulvar cancer. *Gynecologic Oncology*, 34, 263–67.

Thomas, G., Dembo, A., Bryson, S. C. P. *et al.* (1991). Changing concepts in the management of vulvar cancer. *Gynecologic Oncology*, 42, 9–21.

Way, S. (1960). Carcinoma of the vulva. *American Journal of Obstetrics and Gynecology*, 79, 692–7.

References

Cancer of the vagina

Branson, A. N., Dunn, P., Kam, K. C., and Lambert, H. E. (1985). Advice for interstitial therapy of low pelvic tumours—the Hammersmith Perineal Hedgehog. *British Journal of Radiology*, 58, 537–42.

Kuçera, H. and Vavra, N. (1991). Primary carcinoma of the vagina: clinical and histopathological variables associated with survival. *Gynecologica Oncology*, 40, 12–16.

Stock, R. G., Mychalczak, B., Armstrong, J. G. *et al.* (1992). The importance of brachytherapy technique in the management of primary carcinoma of the vagina. *International Journal of Radiation, Oncology, Biology, Physics*, **24**, 747–53.

6

The management of gestational trophoblastic tumours

Introduction

Gestational trophoblastic tumours (GTT) are unique in cancer biology in that the tumours contain paternal genes and are therefore an allograft in the maternal host. They may follow either a normal or abnormal pregnancy.

The most common antecedent pregnancy to a GTT is a complete or partial hydatidiform mole (Table 6.1). Both complete and partial moles remit spontaneously in most cases following evacuation of the uterine cavity. However, either persistent trophoblastic disease or a frank trophoblastic tumour can follow a pregnancy with a complete or partial hydatidiform mole. Therefore, as both types of mole are essentially premalignant conditions, all patients with this diagnosis need to be registered and screened so that the small proportion whose abnormal trophoblast either persists or becomes frankly malignant can receive prompt treatment and elimination of their disease.

A GTT can also occur after a normal pregnancy, with an incidence of between one in 40 000 and 50 000 deliveries. GTT occurring following a full-term pregnancy are always histologically choriocarcinoma and frequently are the highly aggressive variant of this disease, with patients presenting within a few months of delivery with widespread pulmonary and, not uncommonly, cerebral metastases (Tidy *et al.* 1995). Although the incidence of choriocarcinoma occurring following a full-term pregnancy is rare from

Table 6.1 Gestational trophoblastic tumours (GTT): outcome

Antecedent pregnancy	Outcome
Hydatidiform mole	Spontaneous regression
	Persistent trophoblastic disease
	Choriocarcinoma
Normal pregnancy	Choriocarcinoma
Ectopic pregnancy	Placental trophoblastic tumours
Stillbirth	
Spontaneous abortion	

the obstetrician's point of view, in a trophoblastic disease centre such as the Charing Cross Hospital, London, 13 percent of the patients treated had developed a tumour following a full-term pregnancy. Clearly, this possibility needs to be carefully considered in a patient of childbearing years presenting with widespread malignancy.

GTT can occur after ectopic pregnancies, stillbirths, and spontaneous abortions. It is those patients with more obscure obstetric histories that can present major diagnostic problems and awareness of the possibility of a GTT is important.

Pathology and genetics

The term 'gestational trophoblastic disease' is widely used to describe the situation where a woman has had a hydatidiform mole and still has persistently raised human chorionic gonadotrophin (hCG) estimations. Because, in the majority of cases, the disease either remits spontaneously or can be successfully treated without further pathological sampling, it is difficult to say exactly in what proportion of patients their hydatidiform mole modulates to choriocarcinoma. This event probably happens in 3–5 percent of patients who have had a complete hydatidiform mole. When drug-resistant tumour is surgically removed from a patient who has had tissue from a prior mole removed, this is always choriocarcinoma and so there is no doubt that this occurs. The term 'GTT' is used in this chapter to cover all those patients who need chemotherapy for the indications described later under the section Prognostic factors and staging.

Hydatidiform mole

Complete hydatidiform mole forms a multivesicular mass with diffuse hydropic villi and a variable degree of trophoblastic proliferation. There is usually no evidence of a fetus. This conceptus is diploid and androgenetic in origin. Partial moles have been more widely recognized since Szulman and Surti described them in detail in 1978. In the partial mole the hydropic villi tend to be focal and less florid in their development. There is usually evidence of fetal erythrocytes or fetus. Partial moles are triploid conceptuses with two paternal haploid sets of genes and one maternal haploid set.

Invasive hydatidiform mole (complete or partial) is common since molar trophoblast invades the myometrium in most cases, as is confirmed both on ultrasound examination of the uterus and the hCG profile in patients following evacuation of the uterine cavity. Pathologically invasive hydatidiform mole can only be diagnosed when sufficient myometrium is made available to the pathologist either on curetting or by hysterectomy.

Choriocarcinoma

Choriocarcinoma is a tumour composed both of cyto- and syncitio-trophoblastic cells. It is an unusual tumour in that it stimulates virtually no stromal reaction and is therefore essentially a mixture of haemorrhage and necrosis with tumour cells scattered within the mass. Tumour cells can be scanty and present problems of pathological interpretation if the possibility of choriocarcinoma has not been raised. The pathology of choriocarcinoma is reflected in its clinical behaviour with widespread intravascular dissem-ination to lungs, brain, and other sites.

Placental site trophoblastic tumours

Placental site trophoblastic tumours have been recently recognized as a separate entity. These tumours are rare and are composed mainly of cyto-trophoblastic cells and tend to be locally invasive and less widely metastatic than choriocarcinoma (Paradinas and Fisher 1995). The optimal management of patients with placental site trophoblastic tumours is unclear. This is because (i) the tumours are rare and (ii) their biological behaviour does appear to be variable. Where the disease is localized to the uterus, hyster-ectomy is the treatment of choice. A small number of patients treated with intensive chemotherapy initially have achieved complete remission but the chemosensitivity of placental site trophoblastic tumours appears to be quite variable (Dessau *et al.* 1990).

Genetic analysis of GTT

Cytogenetic analysis of complete hydatidiform mole shows that these are paternally derived either by the duplication of the male haplotype following monospermic fertilization of an ovum or, less commonly, by dispermic fertilization of an ovum (Kajii and Omaha 1977; Wake *et al.* 1978). The incidence of a GTT is approximately one thousand times more likely follow-ing a hydatidiform mole than after a full-term pregnancy. One possibility to explain this is that genomic imprinting plays a role in tumorigenesis since the complete mole is androgenetic in origin.

Using microsatellite genetic probes, it is possible to detect paternal genes in tumours to confirm that these are gestational in origin. Some tumours that are morphologically choriocarcinoma, which have been analysed genetically, do not contain paternal genes (Fig. 6.1), and we now recognize that a small number of patients have tumours arising from other sites (e.g. carcinomas of the bronchus, bladder, stomach, colon, and cervix). It is important to recognize that these non-gestational tumours behave differently and, if widely metastatic, are not curable with current therapy. Using these techniques, we have been able to show that a tumour may arise from a prior molar pregnancy with an intervening normal pregnancy (Fisher *et al.* 1992). The polymerase

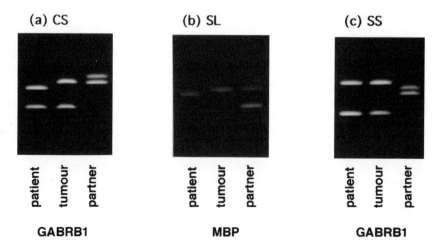

Fig. 6.1 Diagnosis of trophoblastic tumours by PCR analysis of polymorphisms in DNA from parental blood and tumour tissue. GABRBI and MBP represent polymorphic genes examined. (a) a gestational trophoblastic tumour (CS) having both a maternal and paternal contribution to the tumour genome; (b) a gestational trophoblastic tumour (SL) having only a paternal contribution to the tumour genome, suggesting that the tumour originated in a molar pregnancy; (c) a non-gestational tumour (SS) with trophoblastic morphology. In this case only alleles consistent with those in the host are observed.

chain reaction (PCR) is a powerful new technique that potentially allows detailed analysis of GTT from formalin-fixed tissue provided DNA is available from the patient's blood and also from her partner's.

Aetiology, epidemiology, and tumour markers

Aetiology

The cause of GTT remains unknown. If there is a common genetic origin for all GTT, then it is likely that a combination of an abnormality in the paternal genes associated with deletion of a maternal suppressor gene could explain the patterns seen clinically. We know that patients with the andro-genetic conceptus of complete mole have an incidence of persistent tropho-blastic disease/tumour of 8 percent and patients with partial hydatidiform mole have an incidence of persistent disease/tumour of 0.5 percent. This would fit with the situation when there is a relatively common abnormality of the paternal genes in the complete mole where there are no maternal genes to suppress the abnormality, resulting in a relatively high incidence of malignant transformation.

Influence of exogenous hormones

The influence of exogenous hormones on the behaviour of molar tropho-blast is interesting. One explanation for the patient who develops chorio-carcinoma with an intervening normal pregnancy could be that the hormonal surge during the subsequent normal pregnancy stimulates tumour growth from a residue of abnormal tissue persisting after the previous hydatidiform mole (Fisher *et al.* 1992). The effects of exogenous hormones in patients with persistent trophoblastic activity following a hydatidiform mole is an area of considerable controversy. In 1976, Stone *et al.* suggested that women who are exposed to oestrogen and/or progesterone had an increased incidence of malignant sequelae following a molar pregnancy. We have recently analysed the patients treated between 1973 and 1989. Of 8882 patients, 663 (7.5 percent) required chemotherapy and 1384 (15.6 percent) patients received the oral contraceptive. When patients received the oral contraceptive after their hCG had returned to normal, only one of 1049 patients required chemotherapy after that molar pregnancy. This was in contrast with 103 (30.7 percent) of 335 patients who received the oral contraceptive when their hCG was still elevated. Our interpretation of this data is that in the presence of persistent trophoblastic activity following a hydatidiform mole, the disease in a small proportion of these patients can be stimulated by the contraceptive pill, increasing the need for chemotherapy. The reason why this proportion of patients has not been detected in other series in the USA is that our indications for chemotherapy are more conservative and we are prepared to follow patients with elevated hCG for between four and six months before starting chemotherapy. In the US, their policy is to treat patients at eight weeks if their hCG is still elevated. It seems possible that it is the subgroup with more prolonged and persistent trophoblastic activity where disease can be stimulated by the oral contra-ceptive.

Epidemiology

The incidence of complete hydatidiform mole varies in different parts of the world. The best data supporting this is an analysis from Hawaii where in women of Filipino, Japanese, Chinese, and Korean origin the incidence of hydatidiform mole is between 1 per 550 to 1 per 600. This incidence contrasts with the incidence in European immigrants and native Hawaiians, with a frequency of 1 per 1200 live births. Age is also a factor in the incidence of developing complete hydatidiform mole. Where the incidence is standardized as one for women aged 25–29, there is a 6-fold excess in women who become pregnant under 15 years and a 411-fold excess in patients who become pregnant over the age of 50 (Bagshawe *et al.* 1986).

Tumour markers: serial hCG estimations

GTT synthesise a range of hormones, oestrogen, and progesterone and, most importantly, hCG. The monitoring of serial hCG estimations is fundamental to the management of patients with GTT. Although some variants of GTT, such as placental site tumours, produce relatively less hCG than others, it is a universal finding that if a GTT has grown to clinically detectable dimensions, hCG will be detected on a sensitive immunoassay directed against the beta-subunit of hCG. The decay curve of serial hCG estimations of patients on treatment can be used to detect the early development of drug resistance. However, using the initial slope of the hCG decay curve is inaccurate. We have applied regression analysis using the previous six hCG estimations available on a patient to predict whether the decay curve of HCG is going to reach normal at the correct time comparing it to a large database of patients treated successfully. This allows the large database experience of centres, such as the Charing Cross Hospital, to be made available for decision-making on individual patients treated elsewhere, provided they are using a comparable hCG assay (Leaning *et al.* 1992).

Clinical presentation and registration

The most common presentation of a patient with a GTT is a patient with a complete hydatidiform mole with vaginal bleeding towards the end of the first trimester of pregnancy. The patient may also have more nausea and vomiting and be larger-for-dates than for a normal pregnancy. The main differential diagnosis is threatened abortion and ultrasound examination will usually identify both the hydatidiform mole and the absence of a pregnancy. Since the quantity of hCG produced by a normal pregnancy can vary over quite a wide range, the initial hCG estimation is not helpful in differentiating between a pregnancy and a hydatidiform mole.

The initial management of these patients is evacuation of the uterine cavity, usually by suction evacuation. We have analysed the figures for patients registered between 1973 and 1986. For patients who had a single uterine evacuation, only 2.4 percent required chemotherapy. Clearly, those patients having two evacuations probably had more clinical and ultrasound evidence of persistent mole following the initial evacuation. In this group of patients, the incidence of patients requiring chemotherapy rose to 18 percent. A third and fourth evacuation of the uterus is unlikely to prevent the patient from requiring chemotherapy. On these figures our recommendation is an initial diagnostic evacuation and, in selected cases, a second evacuation if there is clinical and ultrasound evidence of a significant amount of trophoblast in the uterus. Further evacuations are probably contra-indicated in most cases.

National follow-up scheme for molar pregnancies

Following the diagnosis of a complete or partial mole, patients in the UK are registered on a national follow-up scheme which was started in 1973 under the auspices of the Royal College of Obstetricians and Gynaecologists and the Department of Health. This service is based in three reference laboratories at Dundee, Sheffield, and London for serial hCG estimations with treatment at London and Sheffield. Seven to 8 percent of patients following a complete hydatidiform mole will require chemotherapy.

The screening and follow-up system for patients with molar pregnancies works extremely well and is highly cost effective. However, patients presenting with GTT after either a full-term pregnancy or an obscure obstetric history, clearly present diagnostic problems. The majority of patients with GTT either in the uterus or elsewhere have irregular vaginal bleeding, due both to the abnormal tissue in the uterus and to the hormones produced by the tumour. A positive pregnancy test in the absence of an intra- or extrauterine pregnancy should alert the gynaecologist to the possibility of a GTT in a young woman of childbearing age. Patients who are on the hydatidiform mole registration scheme who require chemotherapy are selected on the basis of well-established indications for chemotherapy (Table 6.2). The frequency of each indication is shown on the right-hand side of Table 6.2 and a significant proportion of patients have more than one indication for treatment at the time they are admitted.

Prognostic factors and staging

Since 1974 we have used a systematic prognostic scoring system to treat patients (Table 6.3). This separates patients into low-, medium- and high-risk in terms of the intensity of the chemotherapy required to eliminate their

Table 6.2 Indications for treatment for patients with post-molar trophoblastic disease and their incidence (analysis of 552 patients treated between 1982 and 1992)

Indication	Incidence[a] (%)
Rising hCG values	71
Serum hCG above 20 000 units/litre more than 4 weeks after evacuation, because of the risk of uterine perforation	47
hCG in body fluids 4–6 months after evacuation	38
Long-lasting uterine haemorrhage	25
Evidence of metastases in brain, liver, or gastrointestinal tract, or radiological opacities greater than 2 cm on chest X-ray	16
Histological evidence of choriocarcinoma	4

[a] In many patients there was more than one indication for treatment.

Table 6.3 The systematic prognostic scoring system for gestational trophoblastic tumours (in use since 1 August 1993)

Parameter measured	Score 0	1	2	6
Age (yrs)	<39	>39	–	–
Antecedent pregnancy (AP)	Mole	Abortion or unknown	Term	–
Interval from end of AP to chemotherapy at Charing Cross Hospital (mths)	<4	4–7	1–12	>12
hCG (units/litre)	$<10^3$	10^3–10^4	10^4–10^5	$>10^5$
ABO (woman × partner) (blood group)	–	A × O; O × A; O or A × unknown	B × A *or* O; AB × A *or* O	–
No. of metastases	0	1–4	4–8	>8
Site of metastases	Not detected, lungs, vagina	Spleen, kidney	GI tract, liver	Brain
Largest tumour mass (cm)	<3	3–5	>5	–
Previous chemotherapy	0	0	1 drug	≥2 drugs

0–5, low risk; 6–9, medium risk; >9, high risk. GI, gastrointestinal.

disease. This system emphasizes the biological behaviour of the disease rather than the clinical staging. This is more widely used than the current FIGO staging, although the latter now includes hCG concentration, duration of disease, prior chemotherapy, and the presence of a placental site tumour in addition to the clinical staging.

Treatment

Low-risk patients

We have continued to treat low-risk patients with methotrexate and folinic acid. This is a well-tolerated schedule which does not induce alopecia, and the main side-effects are some mucositis and pleuritic chest pain. The disease-specific survival in patients in the low-risk group is 100% but it should be noted that 20 percent of patients need to change from methotrexate because of drug resistance (Fig. 6.2) and a further 5 percent need to change because of toxicity (severe mucositis, pleuritic chest pain, drug-induced hepatitis). These patients have been reported in detail by Bagshawe *et al.* (1989).

Medium-risk patients

In medium-risk patients, we have used drugs in sequence, which has allowed us to introduce etoposide as the initial agent in a group of patients with

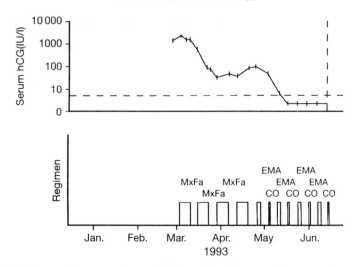

Fig. 6.2 Patient with post-mole trophoblastic disease treated because of rising hCG. Initial response to methotrexate and folinic acid followed by the development of drug resistance is shown by rising hCG concentrations. Prompt remission was induced by the EMA/CO schedule.

already an excellent chance of cure with other agents. Since we introduced etoposide in this context there have been no deaths in the medium-risk category of patients, but a small number have relapsed and have required more intensive therapy (Newlands *et al.* 1986).

The schedules used previously for patients in the medium-risk category required numerous visits to the treatment centre and many days as an inpatient. As longer-term toxicity data has become available with the weekly EMA/CO schedule (Table 6.4) we have largely abandoned the medium-risk schedule and use EMA/CO for patients in this category (Newlands *et al.* 1991).

High-risk patients

Since 1979, in the high-risk patients, we have used the intensive weekly schedule of EMA/CO (Table 6.4). The overall survival was 85 percent in 148 patients treated with this schedule (Newlands *et al.* 1991). There were two subgroups of patients: In the subgroup of 76 patients who had not received prior chemotherapy, the survival was a disappointing 82 percent. Ten of the 14 deaths were due to extensive disease at presentation and death occurred before adequate chemotherapy could be given. None of these 10 patients had presented with a hydatidiform mole and none had been on the follow-up registration scheme. The antecedent pregnancies in this group of patients were full-term pregnancy, stillbirth, or abortion. In the second

Table 6.4 The EMA/CO schedule

Week 1

Day 1

Actinomycin D 0.5 mg iv bolus

Etoposide 100 mg/m^2 iv in 500 ml N saline over 30 minutes

Methotrexate 300 mg/m^2 iv in 1 litre N saline over 12 hours

Day 2

Actinomycin D 0.5 mg iv bolus

Etoposide 100 mg/m^2 iv in 500 ml N saline over 30 minutes.

Folinic acid 15 mg/m^2 orally/iv 12-hourly × 4 doses starting 24 hours after commencement of methotrexate

Week 2

Day 1

Vincristine (Oncovin) 1.4 mg/m^2 iv bolus (max 2 mg)

Cyclophosphamide 600 mg/m^2 iv in 500 ml N saline over 30 minutes

group of 72 patients who had relapsed following previous chemotherapy, the survival was 89 percent. In this group the principal cause of death was the development of drug resistance.

In patients who develop drug resistance, salvage surgery is an important modality. When patients were analysed retrospectively for the effect of surgery in achieving complete remission it was found that the most successful operation in terms of outcome was craniotomy, followed by thoracotomy. Hysterectomy only occasionally resulted in prolonged remission.

Late side-effects, post-treatment fertility, and survival

Second tumour data

Analysis of the entire Charing Cross Hospital series, for the incidence of second tumours following chemotherapy, has recently been carried out (Newlands *et al.* 1995). It is widely recognized that intensive chemotherapy over a prolonged period of time can induce acute myeloid leukaemia.

Controls were age-matched women in the Thames Health regions. There was an overall excess of several tumours: 37 observed, 24.5 expected: relative risk (RR) 1.5 (P = <0.011). There was no significant excess of second tumours in patients only treated with methotrexate and folinic acid. For specific tumours, the risk was significantly increased for myeloid leukaemia RR 16.6 (P = <0.005); adenocarcinoma RR 4.6 (P = 0.005); melanoma RR 4.6 (P = 0.003); and breast cancer treated more than 25 years previously RR 5.8 (P = 0.016). These results emphasize the small but real risk of inducing second tumours and even relatively small doses of etoposide

(1.5 mg/m^2 total dose) can be associated with myeloid leukaemia. It is reassuring that methotrexate and folinic acid do not have this problem and clearly remain the treatment of choice for patients with low-risk disease.

Fertility

After completion of their chemotherapy, patients are followed by serial hCG estimations, initially on serum and urine and in due course on urine alone. At Charing Cross Hospital the recommendation is that patients should not get pregnant for 12 months following chemotherapy to minimize any potential teratogenic effect of chemotherapy. Approximately 90 percent of patients who want to become pregnant following chemotherapy have succeeded and there is no evidence of increase in fetal abnormalities.

Fertility after chemotherapy has been recently summarized by Berkowitz *et al.* (1995). They confirmed that the risk of having a second molar pregnancy is approximately 1 percent. Occasionally, a further GTT can also occur after a subsequent normal pregnancy (Tidy *et al.* 1995). This emphasizes the importance of reconfirming that the hCG returns to normal after every subsequent pregnancy in a woman who has had a prior GTT or trophoblastic disease event. In the five series collected by Berkowitz *et al.* (1995) 77.5 percent of patients had live births after chemotherapy and only 2 percent had fetal abnormalities.

GTT are highly vascular tumours and the very high blood flow through them can now be clearly seen on Doppler ultrasound (Newlands 1995). In the majority of patients this abnormal vascularity regresses after treatment and rarely causes subsequent obstetric problems. However, a small proportion of patients have persistent arteriovenous malformations in the uterus, causing severe vaginal bleeding. As an alternative to hysterectomy in those patients who have not had a family, at Charing Cross Hospital, we have embolized the vascular abnormality with polyvinyl alcohol. With this technique we have had some success in both controlling the bleeding and preserving fertility.

Survival

The original cohort of Charing Cross Hospital patients treated between 1958 and 1973 has a survival of just under 80 percent. The second cohort of patients who were treated between 1974 and 1978 were systematically stratified with the prognostic scoring system shown in Table 6.3, which clearly had an impact on overall survival. The final cohort of 944 patients treated between 1979 and 1992 shows a further incremental improvement in survival which is probably related to the introduction of etoposide and cisplatin for disease resistant to EMA/CO together with better imaging techniques. Computerized tomographic scanning and magnetic resonance imaging has helped in identifying sites for salvage surgery. This current cohort of patients has a survival of 94% with a maximum follow-up of 15 years.

Conclusions

The successful outcome in patients with GTT is due to several factors:

1. The national registration scheme of patients at risk of developing a GTT.
2. The ability to monitor the disease and its response to treatment with serial hCG estimations.
3. The intrinsic biological property of GTT in being very sensitive to a range of chemotherapeutic agents.

References

Bagshawe, K. D., Dent, J., and Webb, J. (1986). Occasional survey: hydatidiform mole in England and Wales 1973–83. *Lancet*, **ii**, 673–7.

Bagshawe, K. D., Dent, J., Newlands, E. S. *et al.* (1989). The role of low dose methotrexate and folinic acid in gestational trophoblastic tumours (GTT). *British Journal of Obstetrics and Gynaecology*, **96**, 795–802.

Berkowitz, R. S. *et al.* (1995). Subsequent pregnancy experience in patients with gestational trophoblastic disease. *Journal of Reproductive Medicine*, **39**, 228–32.

Dessau, R., Rustin, G. J. S., Dent, J. *et al.* (1990). Surgery and chemotherapy in the management of placental site tumor. *Gynecologic Oncology*, **39**, 56–9.

Fisher, R. A., Newlands, E. S., Jeffreys, A. J. *et al.* (1992). Gestational and non-gestational trophoblastic tumours distinguished by DNA analysis. *British Journal of Cancer*, **69**, 839–45.

Kajii, T. and Omaha, K. (1977). Androgenetic origin of hydatidiform mole. *Nature*, **268**, 633–4.

Leaning, M. S., Gallivan, S., Newlands, E. S. *et al.* (1992). Computer system for assisting with clinical interpretation of tumour marker data. *British Medical Journal*, **305**, 804–7.

Newlands, E. S. (1995). Clinical management of trophoblastic disease in the United Kingdom. *Current Obstetrics and Gynaecology*, **5**, 19–24.

Newlands, E. S., Bagshawe, K. D., Begent, R. H. J. *et al.* (1986). Developments in chemotherapy for medium and high risk patients with gestational trophoblastic tumours (1979–1984). *British Journal of Obstetrics and Gynaecology*, **93**, 63–9.

Newlands, E. S., Bagshawe, K. D., Begent, R. H. J. *et al.* (1991). Results with the EMA/CO (etoposide, methotrexate, actinomycin D, cyclophosphamide, vincristine) regimen in high risk gestational trophoblastic tumours, 1979 to 1989. *British Journal of Obstetrics and Gynaecology*, **98**, 550–7.

Newlands, E. S., Rustin, G. J., Lutz, J. M. *et al.* (1995). Chemotherapy for gestational trophoblastic tumours (GTT) may increase the incidence of second tumours and may cause a premature menopause. *Programme and Proceedings of ASCO*, **14**, Abstract 744.

Paradinas, F. J. and Fisher, R. A. (1995). Pathology and molecular genetics of trophoblastic disease. *Current Obstetrics and Gynaecology*, 5, 6–12.

Stone, M., Dent, J., Kardana, A., and Bagshawe, K. D. (1976). Relationship of oral contraception to development of trophoblastic tumour after evacuation of a hydatidiform mole. *British Journal of Obstetrics and Gynaecology*, 83, 913–16.

Szulman, A. and Surti, U. (1978*a*). The syndromes of hydatidiform mole. I: Cytogenetic and morphologic correlations. *American Journal of Obstetrics and Gynecology*, 131, 665–71.

Szulman, A. and Surti, U. (1978*b*). The syndromes of hydatidiform mole. II: Morphologic evidence of the complete and partial mole. *American Journal of Obstetrics and Gynecology*, 132, 20–7.

Tidy, J. A., Rustin, G. J., Newlands, E. S. *et al.* (1995). Presentation and management of choriocarcinoma after nonmolar pregnancy. *British Journal of Obstetrics and Gynaecology*, 102, 715–19.

Wake, N., Takaqi, N., and Sasaki, M. (1978). Androgenesis as a cause of hydatidiform mole. *Journal of the National Cancer Institute*, 60, 51–7.

PART II
Molecular biology

7

Molecular biology of gynaecological cancer

Introduction

Carcinoma can be regarded as a complex failure in cellular homeostasis in which uncontrolled epithelial proliferation occurs in a population of cells that do not communicate normally with the surrounding tissues. As a result, expansion of the tumour cell population occurs, eventually leading to local invasion and distant metastasis.

The concept of carcinogenesis as a genetic disorder involving derangement of the genes which control normal cell growth, differentiation and death is now widely accepted. Within recent years there has been an explosion in the understanding of the complex molecular mechanisms underlying the biological behaviour of tumours. At the centre of this work has been a detailed examination of the genetic basis of cancer.

The genetic code

The genetic code is carried on chromosomes made of deoxyribonucleic acid (DNA) chains composed of nucleotides arranged in a specific sequence unique for each individual. The human genome is made up of 46 chromosomes (22 pairs of autosomal and 1 pair of sex chromosomes). The genes are located at particular sites (loci) on the sequence comprising the chromosome. Each gene carries the information required for the construction of a specific protein molecule.

The DNA is retained in the cell nucleus and protein synthesis takes place on the ribosomes in the cell cytoplasm. Prior to protein synthesis, it is first necessary to make a copy of the DNA, in the form of a messenger ribonucleic acid (mRNA) molecule, by the process of *gene transcription*. The sequences of DNA which contain the coded message (exons) are interspersed between non-coding areas (introns) within the gene. At transcription, a copy of the whole sequence, both exons and introns, is made but the intronic elements are later cut out by the process of splicing. The final mRNA molecule can then carry the message from the nucleus to the ribosome where it is decoded into the amino acid sequence by a process of *translation*. After synthesis, the structure of the protein may be subject to further refinement in the form of post-translational modification. The process by which the information contained in the genetic material of the cell becomes active in the form of functional protein molecules is termed *gene expression*.

Gene expression in normal cells is under rigorous control to ensure that genes are only active, or switched on, when required. Signals from both outside and inside the cell are relayed to the nucleus in order to alter gene expression. In the former case, cell surface receptors receive the initial signal (first messenger) and pass it on to the cell nucleus via a cascade of second messengers by the process of *signal transduction*. Control of gene expression takes place largely at the level of gene transcription mediated by proteins, called transcription factors, which interact with specific DNA sequences called *promoters* or *enhancers*.

Maintenance of the fidelity of the genetic code is of fundamental importance in normal cells. At the time of cell division, complex mechanisms ensure that the DNA copy is an exact reproduction of the original version. There are discrete checkpoints built into the cell cycle to ensure that a cell containing damaged DNA does not duplicate its DNA and proceed to mitosis until all of the damage has been repaired. In addition, proof-reading mechanisms are at work which keep the cellular DNA sequence under constant surveillance allowing rapid detection and repair of damage. Indeed, the presence of excessive or irreparable disruption of the correct DNA sequence will cause activation of mechanisms leading to programmed cell death or *apoptosis* in order to ensure that the errors are not passed on to daughter cells.

Genetic alterations in cancer

In malignant cells, the normal pattern of gene expression is disturbed (Fig. 7.1). This may occur by a number of different mechanisms and, indeed, more than one abnormality is frequently present. In most cases, cancer is thought to arise as a result of a multi-step process in which various genetic alterations are accumulated over a period of time. The genes involved in this process are the *oncogenes*, and/or *tumour suppressor* genes.

Oncogenes

The discovery of cellular oncogenes followed the description of viral genes associated with tumours in animals. The realization that the sequences of the viral genome responsible for tumour development are also present in the cells of organisms as diverse as yeasts, fruit flies, and mammals pointed to the fact that these genes play an essential role in normal cellular functions. In fact, it is thought that the viral oncogenes were initially derived from incorporation of normal cellular oncogenes into viruses, many millions of

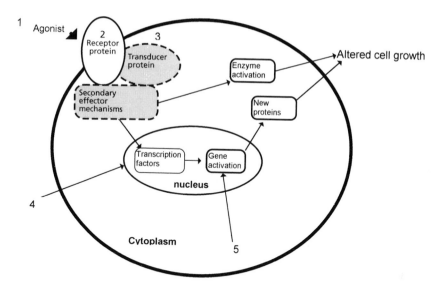

Fig. 7.1 Pathways of cell growth regulation in gynaecological cancer. An overview of the role of oncogenes and tumour suppressor genes in the control of cell growth and proliferation. An agonist acts on the cell, which by use of signalling intermediates such as transducer proteins and secondary effector mechanisms, in turn act on nuclear function. (1) growth factors (eg EGF, TGF-α); (2) receptor tyrosine kinases (eg EGFR); (3) the *ras* group of oncogenes act here; (4) nuclear oncogenes (eg *c-myc*); (5) Tumour suppressor genes (eg p53, retinoblastoma, also mechanism for inactivation by HPV E6 and E7); signalling intermediates.

years ago. The normal cellular genes were called proto-oncogenes to stress the fact that they are only potentially oncogenic.

Mutation of oncogenes results in the formation of a gene product (protein) with enhanced cellular activity. Such mutations are *dominantly acting* since only one of the pair of alleles (see Glossary) needs to be mutated for the cell to manifest the new pattern of gene expression.

The precise cellular functions of normally functioning oncogenes are, as yet, imperfectly understood but their involvement in the cellular machinery controlling growth and development is a recurring theme. For example, abnormalities in genes encoding growth factors or their receptors can lead to the cell receiving excessive growth stimulating signals. Other abnormalities might include those relating to altered control of gene transcription.

Other genes which act as oncogenes are those related to apoptosis such as *bcl2* (an apoptosis suppressor) and *bax* (an apoptosis inducer).

Tumour suppressor genes

Tumour suppressor genes function in a different manner. These genes exert a growth-inhibiting effect in normal cells and give rise to tumours only when their function is lost or reduced. In contrast to the oncogenes, a single normal copy of a tumour suppressor gene is able to maintain normal growth inhibitory function, despite the presence of a mutated copy of the gene on the other chromosome. Therefore, tumours only arise after both normal copies of the gene have been mutated. For this reason, tumour suppressor genes are said to act *recessively*. The classic example of a tumour suppressor gene is the gene for retinoblastoma, *Rb*. Retinoblastomas can occur in an inherited or a sporadic form. In the former case, the patient inherits one abnormal *Rb* gene as a so-called germ-line mutation which is present in every cell in the body. Tumours arise in those cells which lose the function of the remaining allele and so the tumours are multiple and early in onset. On the other hand, sporadic retinoblastomas require the loss of function of both genes by independent events in the same cell and the tumours are seen as solitary cancers with a later age of onset.

Of very considerable interest in the field of solid cancers, including gynaecological malignancies, is the study of the gene *p53*. This gene is located on chromosome 17p and encodes a phosphorylated nuclear protein p53. At a cellular level it is thought to possess a variety of functions including participating in cell cycle control, the maintenance of genomic integrity, and induction of apoptosis in response to DNA damage. Mutations in the *p53* gene are the most common aberrations found in human tumours. Cells containing normal p53 protein (*wild-type protein*) undergo specific pauses in the cell cycle, especially after DNA damage, to allow the cell to restore the genetic sequence to normal. In the presence of mutant p53, these cycle checkpoints are overridden and the cell replicates abnormal DNA sequences and passes them on to the daughter cells. Wild-type p53 is rapidly broken down in normal cells and is usually undetectable. Mutant p53 proteins are more stable, can be detected by immunohisto-chemical stains, and can inhibit the wild type *p53*.

Mechanisms of genetic alteration

Changes in the structure of an individual gene may occur by means of a number of different mechanisms including *point mutations*, *deletions*, *amplifications*, or *translocations*. Alternatively, the structure of the gene may be intact but its regulation may be deranged, for instance, by abnor-malities in transcriptional control, or the gene product may be altered after transcription (e.g. post-transcriptional modification).

Point mutations involve small-scale inaccuracies in the maintenance or reproduction of the genetic sequence—analogous to spelling mistakes. As a result, the amino acid sequence of the synthesized protein is altered depending on the nature and size of the mutation. The *ras* family of onco-genes, *H-ras*, *K-ras*, and *N-ras*, provide the classical example of point muta-tions leading to activation of dominantly acting oncogenes. In this family, mutations in one of only three amino acids at positions 12, 13, and 61 in the protein structure are sufficient to fix the protein in an activated conformation. Point mutations are also common in the tumour suppressor gene, *p53*.

Deletions involve larger-scale losses of the gene and their importance lies in that they can lead to the loss of normal growth control functions. Loss of the second of a pair of tumour suppressor genes often takes this form with deletion of large portions of chromosomal material or even an entire chromosome.

Gene amplification represents the opposite process to gene deletion in that multiple copies of a gene are present, resulting in enhanced synthesis and activity of the encoded protein. The *c-erbB2* oncogene is frequently amplified in breast cancers and in up to one-third of ovarian cancers.

Translocation describes the process whereby part of one chromosome becomes detached from its normal position and joined to another chromosome. This process can bring a gene into an environment where it is subject to different control mechanisms, increasing or decreasing its expression, or can lead to the formation of a new gene by the fusion of parts of two separate genes. The resulting fusion protein may have a novel or an altered function. The Philadelphia chromosome, which is present in chronic myelogenous leukaemia, represents a translocated chromosome in which two genes are brought together to form a new hybrid gene which has an increased activity. In B cell lymphoma there is a 14:18 translocation resulting in overexpression of the *bcl-2* gene.

Abnormalities in the control of gene transcription can lead to enhanced synthesis of gene products in the absence of gene amplification.

Ovarian cancer

Cytogenetic events

Gross cytogenetic alterations are frequently seen in ovarian cancers, with up to two-thirds demonstrating aneuploidy as compared to only one in eight of borderline tumours. There is no consistent pattern of chromosomal alteration and no aberration can be said to be truly specific or diagnostic. However, portions of certain chromosomes (8, 13, 14, 17, 22, and X) are frequently found to be lost from tumours. DNA ploidy has been shown to be an independent prognostic factor in both borderline and invasive epithelial cancers with aneuploid tumours carrying a much poorer prognosis than their diploid counterparts. In addition, the mean S phase fraction, a measure of the number of cells engaged in active DNA synthesis, is higher in malignant than benign ovarian tumours.

Oncogenes

There is a good deal of evidence to implicate a number of oncogenes in the development of ovarian cancers. A cell surface receptor for macrophage colony stimulating factor (M-CSF) encoded by the *c-fms* oncogene is expressed by the majority of ovarian cancers and these same tumours often overexpress M-CSF itself. This provides the tumour with the means of stimulating itself to grow through an autocrine pathway.

Another growth factor which may be active in autocrine growth stimulation is the epidermal growth factor (EGF). As already mentioned, the *c-erbB2 (HER-/neu)* oncogene, which encodes for a version of epidermal growth factor receptor (EGFR), is overexpressed in up to one-third of ovarian cancers and EGFR is expressed by most advanced stage ovarian cancers. EGFR-positive tumours have a worse prognosis than receptor negative tumours.

Tumours suppressor genes

The tumour suppressor gene *p53* is mutated in as many as 50 percent of advanced ovarian cancers. There is some evidence to suggest that this occurs as a late event since few early tumours manifest this abnormality. Recently, two genes, *BRCA1* and *BRCA2*, associated with familial breast and ovarian cancers have been described. Detailed studies of the affected families suggest that *BRCA1* acts as a tumour suppressor gene.

Loss of heterozygosity (LOH)

In ovarian cancer, areas of significant LOH are summarized in Fig. 7.2. Loss of heterozygosity of 30 percent or more is the level accepted as suggestive of a possible site for a tumour suppressor gene.

Endometrial cancer

Cytogenetic events

Cytogenetic abnormalities are not common in endometrial cancers with only 16 percent of tumours exhibiting aneuploidy. Patients with aneuploid tumours are more likely to have aggressive disease with a poor prognosis. Tumour aneuploidy is associated with other markers of poor prognosis.

Oncogenes

Mutations of the *K-ras* oncogene are present in up to 37 percent of cases of endometrial carcinoma. These mutations are present in areas of hyperplasia with atypia adjacent to endometrial cancers but are absent in simple hyperplasia. This finding suggests that *K-ras* mutations may be an early event in the development of the tumour.

Amplification of *c-erbB2* or *c-myc* oncogenes has also been shown to be associated with a poor prognosis. Those tumours which overexpress both oncogenes appear to have a particularly aggressive course.

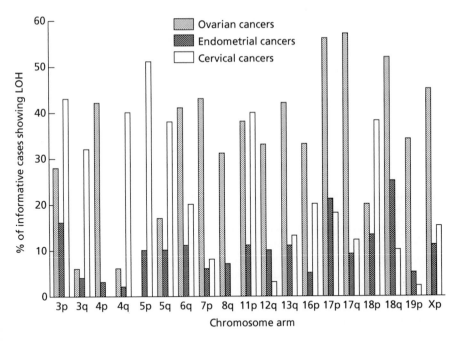

Fig. 7.2 Loss of heterozygosity (LOH) analysis for ovarian, endometrial, and cervical cancers (only chromosome arms showing LOH for one site greater than 30 per cent have been shown (in LOH studies 30 percent of cases showing LOH is accepted as a significant result suggesting a possible site for a tumour suppressor gene).

Tumour suppressor genes

Expression of mutant *p53* occurs most commonly in late stage disease and is associated with a poor prognosis. There is evidence that loss of normal *p53* function occurs as a late event in this situation and may not play an important role in the early development of the tumour.

Loss of heterozygosity (LOH)

A clear consistent pattern of LOH in endometrial cancer (Fig 7.2) has not yet emerged probably due to the small number of tumours studied and the different probes used.

Cervical cancer

Squamous cell cancer of the cervix develops from cervical intra-epithelial neoplasia (CIN) in the transformation zone of the cervix. It is now widely accepted that human papilloma virus (HPV) is the primary causal agent for the development of pre-invasive and invasive cervical cancer.

The papilloma viruses are widely distributed through vertebrates and, although sharing similar genomic organization, are highly species-specific. As the capsid (coating) proteins are antigenically similar, HPVs are divided into genotypes based on the DNA sequence. Over 70 different types of HPV have been identified and they demonstrate significant specificity for anatomic location and the type of lesion produced. Twenty-three types of HPV that infect the anogenital tract have been characterized. HPV DNA can be identified in over 80 percent of women with biopsy-confirmed CIN using techniques such as the polymerase chain reaction (see Glossary). Based on their association with cancer, premalignant lesions or benign epithelial proliferations, the anogenital HPVs have been broadly classified into two different oncogenic groups. Examples of low-risk HPVs associated with condylomata acuminata and the mild forms of CIN are types 6, 11, 42, 43, and 44, whereas high-risk HPVs 16, 18, 31, and 33 are associated with severe CIN and cervical cancers. Low grade cervical lesions are heterogeneous regarding their associated HPV types and may contain more than one type of HPV. High grade lesions are associated with single type HPV infections. HPV 16 is more often seen in squamous cell cancers and HPV 18 is detected more frequently in adenocarcinomas.

HPVs are double-stranded DNA tumour viruses in which the genome is organized into three major regions: (1) two protein-encoding regions; (2) the early and the late gene regions; and (3) a non-coding upstream regulatory region controlling transcription from the early and late gene regions and the production of viral proteins and infectious particles.

The *early* region consists of six open reading frames (ORFs). These are DNA segments, which are transcriptional units capable of encoding for proteins and they are designated *E1, E2, E4, E5, E6* and *E7*. The ORFs encode for proteins synthesized before viral DNA replication. *E6* and *E7* encode for oncoproteins critical for viral replication as well as host cell immortalization and transformation. *E1* and *E2* encode proteins required for extra-chromosomal DNA replication, and completion of the viral life cycle. *E4* gene is involved in the maturation and replication of the virus. *E5* gene interacts with cell membrane receptors for epithelial growth factor and platelet-derived growth factor.

In cervical cancer, HPV DNA is frequently integrated into the host genome but this is often associated with loss or lack of expression of most of the viral genome. However, two of the early genes, *E6* and *E7*, are always retained. Furthermore, the frequent disruption of the *E1* and *E2* genes may release *E6* and *E7* from their usual transcriptional controls. The E6 and E7 proteins interfere with the normal function of *p53* and *Rb* and lead to loss of function. The effect of this is similar to mutation of the respective genes leading to loss of tumour suppressor gene function.

Transforming functions of HPV

Infection of cell lines with HPV 16 and 18 has been shown to lead to alteration in the growth pattern of immortalized cells (cells able to survive in culture after repeated passage) leading to anchorage-independent cell growth. However, infection *prior* to immortalization leads to immortalization alone—the cells are not transformed and are unable to form tumours.

HPV positive cervical cancers and cervical cancer cell lines contain mRNA transcripts from *E6* and *E7*, suggesting that both these genes are required for the transformed phenotype. In human cell *in vitro* systems, *E6* and *E7* alone are not sufficient to transform the cells but following frequent passages after infection the cells exhibit spontaneous changes. This appears to be analogous to the latency between the HPV infection and cervical carcinogenesis *in vivo*.

Cytogenetic events

Numerous structural chromosomal abnormalities have been detected in samples of cervical cancers. Aberrations of chromosome 1 seem relatively common, whilst those of 3, 11, and 17 are less frequent. Similar to the other cancers reviewed, aneuploid tumours of the cervix have a worse prognosis than tumours with a diploid DNA content.

Oncogenes

There have been inconsistent reports of the involvement of oncogenes in the development of cervical cancers. Abnormalities of expressions of *c-myc* and *H-ras* oncogenes have been described.

Tumour suppressor genes

The involvement of the tumour suppressor genes, *p53* and *Rb*, in HPV-related cervical cancers has been described above.

Loss of heterozygosity (LOH)

LOH studies suggest abnormalities at chromosome arms 3, 5, 11 (see Fig. 7.2). In contrast to other solid cancers, loss of heterozygosity of chromosome 17p (the site of the *p53* gene) is unusual in cancers of the cervix. This may be explained by the fact that functional removal of the p53 protein occurs by interaction with the HPV E6 protein.

Vulval cancer

Little has been published with regard to the molecular genetics of vulval cancer. Cytogenetic studies suggest that loss of portions of chromosome arms 10q and 18q are associated with a poor prognosis.

Whilst the frequency of HPV infection in cervical carcinoma is in excess of 80 percent, HPV infection is present in less than 30 percent of vulval cancers, although it is more common in younger patients. Mutant *p53* has been detected in approximately 80 percent of vulval tumours although its clinical significance is, as yet, uncertain.

Gestational trophoblastic disease (GTD)

It has been known for some time that complete hydatidiform moles are diploid with the origin of the genetic material being paternal and that partial hydatidiform moles are usually triploid (69XXY being the most common) with bigenetic parentage. The complete hydatidiform mole containing only paternal DNA results from fertilization of an ovum usually from a duplicated set of 23X chromosomes of a single sperm resulting in a 46XX karyotype. The mechanism of loss of the maternal DNA is unknown. Some complete hydatidiform moles may result from dispermy resulting in a 46XX or 46XY karyotype, the latter being more frequently associated with subsequent clinical sequelae. *p53* mutations do not appear to be significantly involved in GTD. Loss of wild-type *p53* function may contribute to chemoresistance and the finding that *p53* is rarely altered in GTD may explain its marked sensitivity to chemotherapy.

The use of genetic markers is helpful in the clinical setting to determine whether episodes of GTD are from separate fertilization events. The nature of the pregnancy preceding the development of the tumour is important with respect to prognosis and treatment. In a woman who has had multiple pregnancies, it is not always the preceding pregnancy which is causative. The precise origin of the tumour can often be defined by comparing simple repeated DNA sequences, called microsatellites (see Glossary), with archival material and with the father's DNA.

Genetic events in familial cancer

Epidemiological studies have revealed an increased relative risk for ovarian cancer of 1.0–18.2 in women with a family history of this cancer. In 1991, analysis of breast/ovarian cancer families demonstrated linkage to a region of chromosome 17q21 and the *BRCA1* (Breast Cancer 1) gene was identified. The gene frequency of *BRCA1* in the population is 0.0007 and it is responsible for about 50 percent of *familial* ovarian cancer cases but only 2–3 percent of *all* ovarian cancers. *BRCA1* also accounts for 50 percent of inherited breast cancer and two-thirds of families with early onset (less than 45 years of age) breast/ovarian/prostate cancer. Only 58 percent of the documented mutations of BRCA1 occur in these latter families. Mutations of *BRCA1* are found in approximately 10 percent of sporadic ovarian cancers but there is no evidence at present of *BRCA1* abnormalities in the majority of sporadic ovarian cancers.

While the lifetime risk of developing either breast or ovarian cancer by the age of 70 years in a *BRCA1* carrier is greater than 90 percent the data with regard to ovarian cancer risk between different families shows a wide variation, with the majority at a low (26 percent) risk of ovarian cancer by age 70 years and a minority at a high (89 percent) risk. These variations may be explained by different *BRCA1* mutations. Current evidence suggests that most *site-specific* familial ovarian cancers are due to *BRCA1* mutations.

A second gene, *BRCA2* located at 13q12-13, has recently been reported in a series of breast cancer families and some breast/ovarian cancer families not associated with *BRCA1* mutations. In addition to high penetrance genes such as *BRCA1*, it is possible that mutations of genes with a low penetrance but higher prevalence (i.e. relatively low ovarian cancer risk) may account for more cancers than *BRCA1*. As these low penetrance genes will not cause obvious familial aggregation of disease, they will be difficult to find. As the *BRCA1* gene is large and there are multiple different mutations (23 have been identified), the use of *BRCA1* as a simple genetic marker for women at risk is not yet possible.

The hereditary non-polyposis colorectal cancer (HNPCC) syndromes include site-specific hereditary colon cancer HNPCC (Lynch I) syndrome and families with a predisposition to non-polyposis colorectal cancer in association with other cancers including ovarian and endometrial cancer as well as stomach, pancreas, and breast cancer HNPCC (Lynch II) syndrome. Widespread alterations in microsatellites were found in several tumour types including colorectal cancers. The identification of microsatellite instability in tumours from HNPCC patients and that this instability could be reproduced by inactivating mismatch repair genes (*mutS* and *mutL*) suggested that an abnormality of DNA repair genes was responsible for the inherited predisposition to cancer. The basis for the tumour specificity associated with the inherited mutation is unclear since the mismatch repair genes are ubiquitously expressed. In those patients presenting with endometrial cancer, the absence of altered microsatellites in adjacent normal endometrium indicates that the expression of the replication error is limited to neoplastic tissue. The majority of these mutations appear to be acquired prior to clonal expansion suggesting that the underlying genomic instability contributes to the process of carcinogenesis and is not a non-specific consequence of malignant transformation. Microsatellite instability was found in only 17 percent of sporadic endometrial cancers but was present in 75 percent of tumours associated with HNPCC. The lifetime risk of endometrial cancer in individuals with germ line mutations of DNA repair genes is approximately 30 percent.

Cervical and vulval cancer do not show any familial association except in the rare dyskeratosis syndromes.

Management of familial gynaecological cancer

High-risk cases

Women at high risk of gynaecological cancer (10 percent or more lifetime risk) include:

1. women in families with an extensive family history strongly suggestive of one of the familial ovarian cancer syndromes;

2. women with a documented history of ovarian cancer in 2 or more first degree relatives; and

3. women in HNPCC (Lynch II) syndrome families.

Several clinical options are available in management of high-risk cases, these include genetic analysis, screening, chemoprophylaxis, and surgery.

Genetic analysis

If the relevant DNA samples are available (either from blood or archival pathology material) from several other affected family members, it may be possible to perform *linkage analysis* to establish which individual family members have inherited the disease linked chromosome. Mutation analysis is also possible. Both linkage analysis and mutation screening have important ethical and psychological implications which must be considered carefully and discussed with the family members concerned. At present, this form of screening is largely limited to research units but there are a number of centres preparing to offer genetic screening to families as a clinical service.

Screening

The efficacy of screening for sporadic ovarian cancer is unproven. However, in some women with a high risk of ovarian cancer, it is reasonable to commence annual screening about five years prior to the earliest age of onset of cancer in these families with vaginal ultrasonography and/or serum CA125 measurement. Women undergoing ovarian cancer screening should be carefully counselled so that they understand that:

1. Current screening techniques do not detect all cases of ovarian cancer at a preclinical stage.

2. Even when detected preclinically it is not clear whether screen detection has an impact on mortality.

3. There is a significant false positive rate associated with screening which may result in anxiety and unnecessary surgery particularly in premenopausal women.

Breast screening with mammography can start from the mid thirties, although the value of mammography in premenopausal women is controversial. Endometrial screening for women in Lynch II families can be performed by vaginal ultrasonography and endometrial aspiration biopsy but neither of these tests is of proven value. Screening for colorectal cancer and prophylactic surgery for its prevention should be considered.

Chemoprophylaxis

The oral contraceptive pill has been shown to reduce the risk of ovarian cancer in case control studies of sporadic disease and may, therefore, be recommended to women in high-risk families. However, if the mechanism of carcinogenesis in sporadic and familial disease is different, oral contraceptives may not provide the same degree of protection as for sporadic disease. Moreover, it is possible that any benefits may be offset by an increased risk of breast cancer for women in breast/ovarian cancer families.

Surgery

Prophylactic surgery as a primary procedure is justifiable in this group of women on completion of their family after careful confirmation of the family history as well as thorough counselling (bilateral oophorectomy for women at risk of ovarian cancer and total hysterectomy for women at risk of endometrial cancer). The oophorectomy can be performed either by operative laparoscopy or open surgery, as long as all the potentially malignant tissue is completely removed and the patient understands that a full staging procedure would be required if there is evidence of malignancy on histological examination of the specimen. As oophorectomy will usually be performed premenopausally in such cases, long-term hormone replacement therapy (HRT) is essential. The slight increased risk of breast cancer in those taking long-term HRT must be balanced against the benefits in prevention of osteoporosis and cardiovascular disease.

Women at increased risk (2–10 percent lifetime risk)

This group of women includes those with a family history of ovarian cancer which does not include more than one first degree relative. Women in the category of 'increased' but not 'high' risk of ovarian cancer should be reassured that although their risk of ovarian cancer may be increased several-fold it remains relatively small. They should not routinely be offered screening with either CA125 or ultrasound for two reasons. First, an improvement in prognosis for ovarian cancer through detection by screening has not been demonstrated. Second, because the incidence of ovarian cancer in this population is relatively low, the risk of a false positive result resulting in surgical investigation is likely to be more than ten times that of a true positive result (i.e. the positive predictive value of screening is less than 10 percent). The value of screening for women in this group and for those without a family history awaits evaluation in large, well-designed and randomized controlled trials. Oophorectomy should not be recommended as a primary procedure but may be considered as a secondary procedure at the time of surgery for benign disease.

Glossary of common molecular biology terms

Allele Alternative forms of a gene at a given chromosomal site (*locus*)

Amplification Increase in the number of copies of a gene

Apoptosis Active process leading to programmed cell death

Autocrine Growth stimulation induced by the binding of a growth factor secreted by a cell to a receptor in its own cell membrane

Base Adenine, cytosine, guanine, and thymidine—the components of DNA

Chromosome These carry the genetic code made of DNA chains composed of nucleotides arranged in a sequence specific to each individual

Chromosome mapping The assigning of a gene or other DNA sequence to a particular position on a specific chromosome

Cytokine Proteins which act as intercellular signals to co-ordinate the immune response

Deletion Loss of a portion of a chromosome

Exon The base sequence of a gene that carries the information required for protein synthesis

Gene A region of DNA sequence specifying the coding and regulatory sequences for the expression of a protein

Gene expression The process by which the information encoded by a gene is converted into a functional protein. In clinical genetics, the way in which a gene is expressed in an individual

Genome The complete set of genes of an organism and the intervening DNA sequences

Genotype The genetic constitution of an individual, usually at a particular site

Growth factor Proteins that bind to receptors on the surface of cells and modify their growth

Growth factor receptor Proteins embedded in the cell membrane with an extracellular receptor region and an intracellular signalling region. The receptor can be activated by the growth factor

Heterozygote An individual with two different alleles at the same locus on each of a pair of chromosomes. A heterozygote who has a dominant disease gene and one normal gene will be affected by the disease; one who has a recessive disease gene and a normal gene will be a carrier

Homozygote An individual who has two identical alleles at the same locus on a pair of chromosomes

Intron Transcribed portions of the DNA sequence that do not contain coding information for protein synthesis

Linkage The tendency for genes lying close together on the same chromosome to be inherited together

Locus Site on a chromosome

Loss of heterozygosity Loss of one allele at a chromosomal locus, followed by deletion of the remaining locus leading to homozygosity

mRNA Messenger RNA formed by the transcription of DNA

Microsatellites Repeated DNA sequences in tandem. They are short segment repeats of 2–4 nucleotides common within introns and show pronounced polymorphism useful for: (i) gene mapping and linkage analysis; (ii) markers of loss of heterozygosity; and (iii) as a diagnostic tool for detecting tumour cells in histologically unremarkable specimens

Mutation A change in DNA sequence. This can range from an alteration in a single base (e.g. sickle-cell haemoglobin) to loss or gain of chromosomal material (e.g. the Philadelphia chromosome in chronic myeloid leukaemia)

Northern blotting Laboratory technique for locating RNA sequences

Nucleotide A subunit of nucleic acids (DNA, RNA) consisting of a base, a sugar, and a phosphate

Oncogene A gene whose product can cause cancer by stimulating abnormal cell growth and excessive proliferation

Open reading frames DNA segments which are transcriptional units capable of encoding for proteins

Phenotype The physical characteristics of an individual resulting from the interaction of its genotype with environmental factors

Polymerase chain reaction This is a way of 'amplifying' or making multiple copies of any piece of nucleic acid. It allows amplification of any gene sequence

Polymorphism The existence, in a population, of two or more relatively common alleles at a genetic locus. It is a *variation* in the sequence of the gene that tracks with the gene and is not a mutation

Promoter/enhancer DNA sequences that act as control points for DNA transcription

Proto-oncogene A gene that normally regulates cell growth and proliferation but which can cause cancer when mutated

Reverse transcription DNA synthesis from RNA templates. It occurs naturally in retroviruses and is used to synthesize DNA in the laboratory

Southern blotting Laboratory technique for detecting DNA sequences

Splicing Process by which intronic sequences are removed from initial RNA transcript to form messenger RNA

Transcription The synthesis of RNA from its corresponding DNA sequence

Transcription factor Specific regulatory proteins that control gene expression by switching genes on and off

Translation Production of a protein from mRNA code

Translocation Exchange of DNA material between chromosomes

Tumour suppressor genes (TSG) A gene which normally slows growth and proliferation. Abnormalities of TSGs can lead to uncontrolled cell replication and so to malignancies

Western blotting A laboratory technique for detecting proteins

Further reading

Jacobs, I. and Lancaster, L. (1996). The molecular genetics of sporadic and familial epithelial ovarian cancer. *International Journal of Gynecological Caner*, **6**, 337–55.

Jeyarajah, A., Oram, D. H. and Jacobs, I. (1996). Molecular events in endometrial carcinogenesis. *International Journal of Gynecological Cancer*, **6**, 425–38.

Park, T.-W., Fujiwara, H., and Wright, T. C. (1995). Molecular biology of cervical cancer and its precursors. *Cancer*, **76**, 1902–13.

PART III
Main methods of treatment

8

Surgery

Introduction

Surgery plays a key role in the diagnosis, staging, and therapy of gynaecological malignancy.

Diagnosis

In order to confirm a diagnosis of gynaecological malignancy, surgery is
carried out to obtain the histological material needed. This may vary from a
biopsy to removal of an entire organ such as the ovary.

Staging

Staging of gynaecological cancers is essential both for planning appropriate
treatment and for comparing treatment results from different centres. The
FIGO system is the one most frequently used (see Chapter 1, p. 3), and
details of the FIGO system for each tumour can be found in the chapters on
these malignancies. This staging system is based on the *surgical* and *pathological* findings in ovarian, endometrial, vaginal and vulval cancers but for
cancer of the cervix FIGO staging is *clinical* and is dependent on careful
examination of the pelvis, whilst the woman is under a general anaesthetic.

Treatment

Surgery plays an important role as primary therapy in gynaecological
cancer. The aim is the complete removal of the tumour with a margin of
normal tissue. In advanced disease this is not possible and surgery may then
be combined with, or replaced by, other treatment modalities. For example,
radiotherapy may be used before or after surgery in vulval cancer and
chemotherapy is usually given post-operatively for epithelial ovarian cancer.
In advanced cancer of the cervix surgery is replaced by radiotherapy.

Less frequently, surgery is used as a salvage treatment in some cases of
residual disease after radiotherapy or chemotherapy or in recurrent disease.
It also plays a part in palliation, such as stoma formation for bowel
obstruction.

In this chapter, various procedures relating to gynaecological oncology
are detailed. The indications for each procedure are given elsewhere in the
book.

Minor procedures

Examination under anaesthetic (EUA)

This procedure is performed under general anaesthesia, as its name implies. It is used for the staging of cervical cancer, assessment of disease progression, and planning of major surgery.

The woman is placed in the lithotomy position. The perineum is inspected and then the genital area and vagina are cleaned with aqueous antiseptic solution. If indicated, a cystoscopy (an endoscopic examination of the bladder) will be done first. Then the procedures relating to the cervix and uterus are performed. Finally, an anorectal examination is carried out.

The pelvic examination should include bimanual and bidigital examination. The bimanual examination is performed as follows: the labia are gently separated and the lubricated index and middle fingers of one hand are inserted into the vagina. The other hand is placed on the lower abdomen and the pelvic organs are palpated between both hands in a systematic fashion. Information regarding the vagina, cervix, uterus, and adnexae is obtained from the examination. The bidigital examination, with the index finger in the vagina and the middle finger in the rectum, allows palpation of the rectovaginal septum, the pouch of Douglas, uterosacral and cardinal ligaments (parametrium), pelvic side wall, and rectum. At the end of the examination, the doctor should be able to describe the size, shape, and interrelation of the pelvic organs in an ordered anatomical fashion and detail the presence of masses or other abnormalities.

Hysteroscopy and endometrial biopsy

Hysteroscopy (using an endoscope to examine the uterine cavity) has largely replaced the blind sampling of the endometrium by dilatation and curettage (D&C). The procedure is usually performed under general anaesthetic although it can be done in the outpatient setting with either no or only local anaesthesia (paracervical block). Using a Sims speculum, the vagina and cervix are visualized. The anterior lip of the cervix is grasped with a tenaculum (e.g. Vulsellum tenaculum, a type of tissue-holding forceps). This stabilizes the cervix and uterus during the procedure as well as straightening the cervical canal allowing easy passage of the instrument. Usually, the diagnostic hysteroscope (4 mm diameter) will pass without prior dilatation of the cervix. Saline irrigation is used in diagnostic procedures although carbon dioxide insufflation can be used in the outpatient setting, and non-conducting solutions (glycine) are used when operative hysteroscopy is performed. The tubal ostia are identified and any abnormality, such as polyps, fibroids, or carcinoma, is noted. Directed biopsy of this abnormality can be performed as required. If no focal lesion needs biopsy then an endometrial sample for histology can be obtained using a small curette following the hysteroscopy. Dilatation of the cervical canal beyond Hegar 6 (the diameter of the graded dilators measured in millimetres) for diagnostic reasons is rarely needed.

Cervical biopsy (including cone biopsy)

Any abnormality of the cervix (other than a frank carcinoma of the cervix), whether detected by cytological surveillance or suspected by clinical examination, should be assessed by colposcopy. This involves an examination of the cervix using a low power microscope and various solutions (3–5 percent acetic acid and Lugol's iodine) which highlight epithelial abnormalities. Colposcopic directed biopsy of cervical abnormalities is performed as an outpatient using punch biopsy forceps.

Cone biopsy

A cone biopsy (Fig. 8.1) is required either for treatment for pre-malignant or early (superficial invasive) disease of the cervix or as an aid for diagnosis, when the colposcopic examination is inadequate or incomplete. A cone-shaped piece of the cervix containing the transformation zone is removed and sent for pathological examination.

Excisional techniques for treating pre-malignant lesions of the cervix are considered to be superior to ablation as they allow histological analysis. Excisional techniques include scalpel (a 'cold knife' cone usually performed under general anaesthetic), diathermy (LLETZ, large loop excision of the

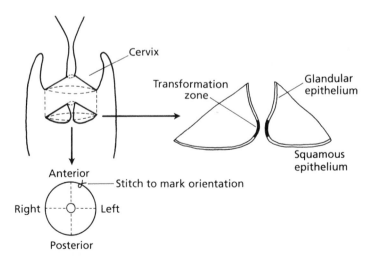

Fig. 8.1 A cone biopsy must include all the transformation zone. It is often marked to allow orientation of the specimen by the pathologist.

transformation zone), and laser. Ablative techniques include laser, radical electrocoagulation diathermy (under general anaesthetic), cold coagulation (a misnomer as the 'Semm cold coagulator' operates at 100°C), and cryotherapy. Due to the ease of use, low cost, and acceptability of the treatment, LLETZ (or *Loop Electrocautery Excisional Procedure*, LEEP, in the USA) has become the predominant form of treatment, especially in the outpatient setting using a cervical block for anaesthesia. Although lasers (usually the carbon dioxide laser) are less frequently used in pre-malignant disease of the cervix and genital tract, there is a role for their use in extra-cervical intra-epithelial neoplasia in the vagina (VAIN), vulva (VIN), and anus (AIN).

Laparoscopy

Laparoscopy (the endoscopic inspection of the abdomen) can be used for diagnostic purposes or for operative procedures. It is usually performed under general anaesthetic and often as a day case procedure. The patient is placed supine with the legs supported at 45 degrees with the stirrups. A pelvic examination is performed, the bladder is emptied via a catheter, and a uterine manipulator (e.g. Spackman cannula) is attached to the cervix. The abdominal cavity is inflated with carbon dioxide via a hollow needle (Verres needle). When the pneumoperitoneum is sufficient to protect the viscera from the sharp trocar, the telescope is introduced at the umbilicus. Nowadays, most laparoscopies are performed using a camera system and the view is seen on a television monitor. The abdominal and pelvic contents are inspected in a standard fashion which is documented. Manipulation of the abdominal organs is facilitated by the use of instruments inserted through further ports. The laparoscope gives excellent views due to its magnification as well as its access in the pelvis and upper abdomen. There is an increasing use of operative laparoscopy in gynaecology but its role in gynaecological oncology has yet to be determined. Pelvic and para-aortic lymph-adenectomy and laparoscopically assisted hysterectomy (both simple and radical) are possible but as yet unevaluated.

Major pelvic surgery

Pre-operative care

For radical surgery, bowel preparation is usual as the bowel should be mechanically clean if intestinal surgery is required and also it is more comfortable for the patient in the first few post-operative days. Blood is cross-matched for radical surgery. Prophylactic antibiotics covering aerobic and anaerobic bacteria (e.g. a cephalosporin and metronidazole) are given for both abdominal and vaginal operations as these reduce the likelihood of wound and vault infections. Prophylaxis against thrombosis (e.g. subcutaneous heparin) is also important as the patient is at an increased risk due to malignancy and pelvic surgery. Appropriate informed consent is obtained. Histological confirmation of the diagnosis is important prior to radical surgery (although not always possible in ovarian cancer).

Laparotomy

Laparotomy allows access to the abdominal and pelvic organs. In a woman with a pelvic malignancy (or suspected malignancy as in the case of ovarian cancer), the abdomen is opened via a midline incision. This midline incision is often extended above the umbilicus to allow free access to the whole abdomen, especially useful in ovarian cancer. Paramedian incisions are rarely used nowadays as the use of appropriate suture material and techniques have reduced the risk of dehiscence and hernia formation. In certain cases, such as early cancer of the cervix where only a pelvic lymphadenectomy and radical hysterectomy are performed, a low transverse incision (Pfannensteil) may be sufficient. This type of incision has the advantage of giving a strong scar and a good cosmetic result but gives limited access to the upper abdomen.

Once the incision has been made, any free fluid present is aspirated for cytological examination for the presence of malignant cells. In suspected ovarian and endometrial cancer, abdominal and pelvic peritoneal washings are carried out using warm saline.

The abdominal and pelvic contents are then examined carefully and systematically including the diaphragm, liver, stomach, large and small bowel, and mesentery. The retroperitoneum over the aorta, the inferior vena cava and major pelvic vessels are palpated for lymphadenopathy. Palpation will not detect micrometastases and enlarged nodes do not always contain cancer. In UK practice, the routine use of para-aortic and pelvic lymphadenectomy for staging gynaecological cancer, as suggested by FIGO, is not common.

Closure of a midline incision is performed using a non-absorbable (nylon) or slow-dissolving monofilament (PDS) looped suture, which passes through all layers of the abdominal wall (mass-closure technique). There are reduced rates of abdominal dehiscence and incisional hernia with this method of closure. The transverse incision is less likely to be the cause of incisional hernia.

Hysterectomy

The removal of the uterus and the cervix constitutes a total hysterectomy. This may be performed *abdominally* (total abdominal hysterectomy, TAH) or *vaginally*. A *simple* hysterectomy relates to the plane of removal, close to the uterus and on the cervix, rather than the ease of surgery. The removal of both the ovaries and fallopian tubes is called a bilateral salpingo-oophorectomy (BSO) (Fig. 8.2). A *radical* hysterectomy is a much bigger operation removing the uterus and cervix with a cuff of surrounding tissue (Fig. 8.3). The various types of hysterectomy are detailed in Table 8.1.

The hysterectomy is performed by dividing the blood supply from the ovarian and uterine vessels, the supports of the uterus (uterosacral and cardinal ligaments), and the peritoneal coverings (the round and broad ligaments, uterovesical fold, and pouch of Douglas). In the abdominal procedure, the BSO is performed first, if indicated, by dividing the

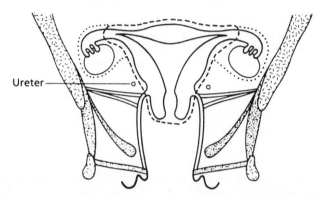

Fig. 8.2 A simple total hysterectomy. The excised tissues include the body of the uterus and the cervix. As the vaginal incision is made through the fornices, only a minimal amount of the vagina is removed. The ureters are undisturbed as the line of incision is close to the cervix. The fallopian tubes and ovaries are removed as a bilateral salpingo-oophorectomy.

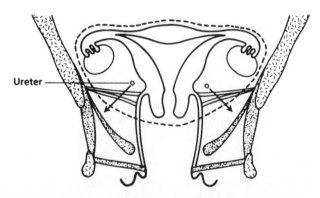

Fig. 8.3 A radical hysterectomy in which the ureters are mobilized to allow wide excision of the cervix, uterus, and surrounding parametrium. The uterine arteries are divided at their source from the internal iliac artery. The cardinal ligaments and a vaginal cuff (upper third) are also removed. The ovaries can be preserved.

Table 8.1 Types of hysterectomy

Subtotal hysterectomy   Removal of the uterus alone is rarely used in modern oncology. An increasing number of gynaecologists using minimal invasive surgery are using a supracervical (subtotal) hysterectomy having removed the transformation zone and glandular tissue from the cervix in benign conditions.

Total abdominal hysterectomy +/− bilateral salpingo-oophorectomy (TAH +/− BSO)   Also known as a simple hysterectomy. The removal of the uterus and cervix with a minimum of the surrounding parametrium and paracervical tissue.

Extended hysterectomy   The complete removal of the uterus and cervix including a cuff of vaginal tissue without significant disturbance of the ureters.

Radical abdominal hysterectomy (Wertheim).   Removal of the cervix and surrounding tissues from the bladder anteriorly to the rectum posteriorly with the pelvic side wall laterally and a cuff of vagina (approximately upper third or two cm beyond the tumour). At the same operation, a bilateral pelvic lymphadenectomy is performed. This is a Rutledge type 2–3 radical hysterectomy (Piver *et al.* 1974). The removal of the Fallopian tubes and ovaries is optional.

Vaginal hysterectomy   Removal of cervix and uterus by the vaginal route, see **Total abdominal hysterectomy.**

Laparoscopic vaginal hysterectomy   A technique allowing the assessment of the peritoneal cavity and allowing division of the pedicles and any adhesions under direct vision. There are variations as to how much surgery is performed laparoscopically and how much is performed vaginally.

Radical vaginal hysterectomy (Schauta)   The radical removal of the cervix with an appropriate margin of normal tissue. A muscle cutting vaginal incision (Schuhardt) can be used for ease of access. It is not possible to remove the lymph nodes via the vaginal route and the pelvic lymphadenectomy can be done either transperitoneally using laparoscopic techniques or via the retroperitoneum.

Rutledge classification of extended hysterectomy for cervical cancer (Piver *et al.* 1974)

Class 1   Ensures removal of all cervical tissue: also called extrafascial hysterectomy

Class 2   Modified radical hysterectomy removing the medial half of the cardinal and utero-sacral ligaments. The uterine vessels are divided medial to the ureter

Class 3   The classical Wertheim–Meig's radical hysterectomy. *Aim:* the wide radical excision of the parametrial and paravaginal tissue. The ureter is dissected down to the bladder. The uterosacral ligaments are divided at their origin and the cardinal ligaments are divided at the pelvic wall

Class 4   More radical than class 3. The ureter is completely dissected from the pubovesical ligament, the superior vesical artery is sacrificed and 75% of the vagina is removed. Rarely used except for surgically resectable recurrences

Class 5   The removal of a central recurrence involving the ureter or bladder. In the UK, an exenteration would be used

infundibulopelvic ligament containing the ovarian vessels. To ensure that the ureter, which is usually situated relatively close on the pelvic side wall, is not included in this pedicle, the round ligament is opened and the ovarian vessels are clearly identified above the ureter. The uterovesical fold of

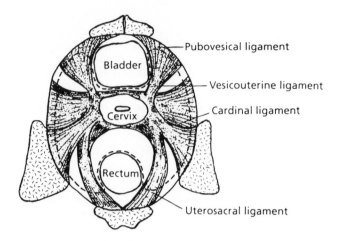

Bladder

Pubovesical ligament

Vesicouterine ligament

Cervix

Cardinal ligament

Rectum

Uterosacral ligament

Fig. 8.4 The ligaments supporting the uterus at the level of the cervix.

peritoneum is divided and the bladder reflected off the cervix. The uterine vessels are identified, clamped, divided, and ligated. Further tissue is divided (and ligated) close to the cervix including the uterosacral and the cardinal ligaments (Fig. 8.4). The vagina is opened and the uterus and cervix are removed. The edges of the vagina are oversewn to secure haemostasis. In cervical disease, it is recommended that the vault is oversewn and left open so as not to bury any recurrence of CIN at the vaginal margin.

Vaginal hysterectomy

The vaginal hysterectomy is performed in a similar manner but in reverse order. Following the division of the uterosacral and cardinal ligaments, the uterus will descend into the vagina with ease. The uterine vessels can then be identified, clamped, divided, and ligated. If required, the ovaries may be removed vaginally with or without laparoscopic assistance.

Extended hysterectomy

An extended hysterectomy is a term frequently used in relation to surgery for women with endometrial carcinoma. This indicates a simple hysterectomy (see p. 159 for distinction between simple and radical hysterectomy) where attention is paid to removing the complete cervix including some of the vagina (i.e. the clamps used after the uterine artery are applied in the parametrium rather than on to the cervix). Care has to be taken to avoid the ureter, which lies close to the uterine vessels.

Radical hysterectomy and bilateral pelvic lymphadenectomy

This operation is the treatment of choice for early carcinoma of the cervix.

The operation consists of the removal of the central tumour and the draining lymph nodes: the radical hysterectomy removing the cervix containing the tumour with an adequate cuff of normal material (the parametrium and paracolpos) and the bilateral pelvic lymphadenectomy. The radical hysterectomy was first described in Vienna at the turn of the century by Wertheim, and was then modified by Meigs who added the systematic pelvic lymphadenectomy, hence the procedure is often known as a Wertheim's or Wertheim–Meig's operation.

The lymphadenectomy can be done either at the beginning of the operation or after the uterus has been removed. The side wall is opened and the external iliac vessels are identified. The lymphatic tissue adjacent to the external iliac vessels is stripped from the circumflex iliac vein distally up to and including tissue around the common iliac vessels. Care is taken to preserve the genito-femoral nerves. Then the lymphatic tissue is removed from the obturator fossa with careful preservation of the obturator nerve. The ureter is identified and the internal iliac lymphatic tissue is removed. Haemostasis is obtained with diathermy and titanium haemostatic clips (Ligaclips). Some surgeons send the lymphatic tissue as separate samples, as involvement at multiple sites carries a significantly poorer prognosis.

If the ovaries are to be preserved then the ovarian ligament is divided and ligated. If the ovaries are to be removed, the infundibulo-pelvic ligament is ligated and divided. The ureter is dissected free from its surrounding tissue and the uterine artery is ligated and divided at its origin on the anterior branch of the internal iliac artery. The ureteric tunnel is opened and the ureter dislocated medially and traced down towards the bladder. The utero-sacral and cardinal ligaments (Fig. 8.4) are divided on the rectum and near the pelvic side wall, respectively. This tailored approach, popular in the UK, is classified between Rutledge 2 and 3 procedures (Piver *et al.* 1974; see also Table 8.1). The vagina is divided approximately two centimetres below the cervix and its tumour.

Closed suction drains are used if there has been significant bleeding but routine drainage of the pelvic sidewall to reduce lymphocyst formation and ureteric fistula formation is being questioned. The bladder is kept on continuous catheter drainage for 7–10 days. This is because the autonomic nerve supply to the bladder is affected by the posterior dissection around the uterosacral ligaments and, as a result of the surgery, there is significant oedema around the bladder base. This bladder drainage reduces the risk of fistula formation.

Radical vaginal hysterectomy

Treatment of the draining lymph nodes has been accepted practice in the surgical management of cervical cancer for the past 60 years, and has been the rationale for the abdominal approach for hysterectomy. The radical vaginal hysterectomy (Schauta operation see Table 8.1) removes the primary tumour with an adequate margin of normal tissue and this can be facilitated using a muscle cutting episiotomy (Schuhardt's incision). The primary cure rate is similar to that of the radical abdominal operation but with reduced morbidity. The vaginal approach has not been widely used because of the lack of the necessary expertise and because of the necessity of treating the pelvic lymph nodes which was usually performed by the extra-peritoneal approach requiring extra incisions. However, there is now renewed interest in the radical vaginal procedures with the advent of laparoscopic surgery. Using laparoscopic surgery a pelvic and, if necessary, a para-aortic lymphadenectomy can be performed. Other modifications of surgical technique are also being reported and the long-term results of all these new variations await evaluation.

Radical hysterectomy for endometrial cancer

Radical hysterectomy for endometrial cancer is seldom used. In stage II disease, where there is cervical involvement, some clinicians suggest that a radical hysterectomy should be performed because there may be difficulty in defining pre-operatively those cases of endocervical adenocarcinoma spreading up to the uterus from those women with an endometrial adeno-carcinoma spreading down to the cervix.

Cytoreductive surgery

Cytoreductive surgery is carried out for advanced ovarian cancer. The aim is to remove the tumour completely or to reduce its bulk leaving residual disease smaller than one centimetre (1 cm) at its largest diameter. The situation with either no residual tumour or deposits smaller than 1 cm following surgery is termed 'optimal cytoreduction'. Whether this is attainable depends on the inherent biology of the tumour as well as on the surgeon's skill and training. Although optimal cytoreduction is possible in about two-thirds of patients, cytoreductive surgery must be attempted by an appropriately trained surgeon because it is not possible to determine, pre-operatively, which cases will be successful.

Cytoreductive surgery is most commonly carried out as *primary surgery* at the initial staging but is also performed in women with unresectable or unresected, but biopsy proven, disease who have responded to three or four cycles of chemotherapy. This is known as *interval* or *intervention surgery* and is followed by further chemotherapy.

Secondary surgery includes all the other aspects such as the second-look procedure, secondary cytoreductive, and palliative surgery. Women with a late relapse (more than 1–2 years following primary treatment) may occasionally benefit from further surgery prior to further chemotherapy. *Second look surgery* was performed in women who had achieved a clinical complete response following primary surgery and adjuvant chemotherapy. No survival advantage has been demonstrated using this surgery and the procedure is currently not used in the UK.

Procedure for cytoreductive surgery

Following infracolic omentectomy, if it is apparent that there is little residual tumour in the upper abdomen (i.e. either no disease or nodules less than 1 cm), then it would be appropriate to proceed to a radical oophorectomy. As the tumour tends to remain intraperitoneally, the operative technique makes use of the retroperitoneal plane. This allows the clear identification of the important structures (ureters and blood vessels) where they are not obscured by tumour. The peritoneum is opened above the pelvic brim and the ureters and pelvic vessels are dissected free under direct vision. Using the pre-sacral plane, the tumour mass in the pouch of Douglas is elevated and a hysterectomy is performed. The uterine vessels are ligated laterally. A rectosigmoid resection may be necessary to remove the tumour mass although direct reanastomosis is usually possible. This radical approach involving bowel resection is only appropriate when optimal cytoreduction is achieved, although its value with regard to survival has recently been questioned (Potter *et al.* 1991).

Lymphadenectomy in ovarian cancer

The lymph drainage from the ovary passes to both the pelvic lymph nodes and to the para-aortic lymph nodes around the renal vessels. Lymphadenectomy must, therefore, include both these areas. The value of pelvic and para-aortic lymphadenectomy with regard to survival is being reviewed in an international trial. In patients with presumed early disease it is known that a significant number of cases have occult micrometastases (Young *et al.* 1983) but it is rare for lymphadenectomy to be carried out in the UK.

Vulval surgery

Minor procedures

The use of combined clinics between dermatologists and gynaecologists has led to better management of vulval conditions. A number of these conditions are pre-malignant and as the distinction between pre-invasive and early invasive vulval and perineal disease can be difficult adequate biopsies should be taken. Often, these biopsies can be done in the outpatient setting under local anaesthetic. Occasionally, wider excision biopsies are required and are performed under general anaesthetic. The use of a simple vulvectomy, the removal of the superficial skin of the vulva, is rarely indicated (Fig. 8.5). It is easier to remove the abnormal areas as they occur

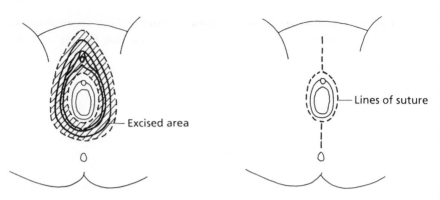

Fig. 8.5 The area of skin removed in a simple vulvectomy and the suture lines used to close the defect.

and have careful follow-up rather than remove excessive areas of normal tissue. Apart from the psychological morbidity of the procedure, the conditions for which a simple vulvectomy are appropriate tend to recur and may return, even on grafted skin.

Radical surgery

Surgery for vulval cancer is becoming centralized to specialized centres. One of the consequences has been the modification of older techniques leading to more tailored surgery for each patient. Until recently standard radical vulvectomy included the complete removal of the vulva and bilateral inguino-femoral lymph nodes using the butterfly incision. In those cases where the nodes were considered to be positive the lymphadenectomy was extended to include the pelvic nodes. Although giving good results in terms of 5-year survival, the high risk of complications, such as wound dehiscence and thrombosis, resulting from this extensive surgery in an elderly population, was unacceptable.

Surgery for the primary tumour now consists of wide excision with an adequate margin of normal tissue (usually 1 cm) where possible. While removal of the complete vulva is no longer an absolute requirement, in some cases plastic surgery techniques, such as rotation flaps or myo-cutaneous grafts, may be required in order to obtain skin closure without tension.

If the lesion is less than 1 millimetre deep (superficial invasion), vulval excision without lymphadenectomy is sufficient treatment. In all other cases, an ipsilateral or bilateral inguinal and superficial femoral lympha-denectomy should be performed. At present, pre-operative investigations are not sufficiently sensitive to detect lymph node metastases. The patho-logical status of the lymph nodes is part of the FIGO staging and gives important prognostic information (see Chapter 5, p. 101).

Separate incisions are made in the inguinal region to remove the inguinal and superficial femoral lymph nodes (see Fig. 5.2, p. 106). The routine division of the long saphenous vein is part of the classic description of the lymphadenectomy but preservation of the vessel may have some benefit in reducing the incidence of leg lymphoedema. The opening of the cribriform fascia to remove the deep femoral lymph nodes is rarely indicated. The incision and more 'tailored' removal of tissue contrasts with the radical block dissection used in melanoma.

Pelvic lymph nodes are not removed. If the inguinal nodes contain metastatic deposits, the pelvic nodes are treated by radiotherapy which has been found to be more effective than surgery (Holmesley *et al.* 1986).

Surgery for recurrent cancer

Exenteration

Recurrent pelvic cancer can sometimes be amenable to surgery both for cure and for palliation. This major surgery may involve removing the bladder (*anterior exenteration*), rectum (*posterior exenteration*), or both (*total exenteration*). Even at major centres, exenterative surgery is not common. In ovarian and endometrial cancer, this type of surgery is rarely indicated but in cervical cancer, an isolated central pelvic recurrence can be removed by surgery with 5-year survival rates of around 50 percent (Shepherd *et al.* 1994). In vulval cancer, exenteration may be considered when the tumour has involved the anal sphincter, although the use of pre-operative radiotherapy may 'downgrade' the tumour involvement allowing sparing of a functional sphincter.

Urinary diversion and colostomy

Diversion of the urinary or faecal stream is sometimes required in the management of gynaecological cancer (e.g. if a fistula occurs). The urinary tract can be replaced either by a conduit (either ileal or colonic) or a continent diversion. The ileal conduit is formed from an isolated loop of terminal ileum which forms a wet stoma between the ureters and abdominal wall. The alternative continent diversion which does not need an abdominal appliance is not usually offered in the palliative case as it requires more complicated surgery with more associated problems. All continent procedures use detubularized bowel to construct a low pressure reservoir which has a spout with an antireflux mechanism through which the catheter is passed to void the neo-bladder.

The faecal stream can be diverted by a variety of methods. The aim is to re-anastomose the bowel to restore continuity and this is often securely achieved using stapling devices. However, re-anastomosis is not always possible, especially of irradiated bowel which heals poorly due to a compromised blood supply. In such cases, colostomies, either end or loop, and ileostomies may be needed. In those cases of bowel obstruction secondary to gynaecological cancer, internal bypass may be appropriate, but often a stoma or medical management are all that is possible.

Complications of surgery

These can be detailed in chronological order relating to problems occurring at the time of surgery, in the immediate post-operative period (i.e. up to two weeks after surgery), and later. Complications may also be related to surgery in general (e.g. thromboembolism) or to the procedure directly (e.g. damage to the ureter during radical hysterectomy).

Complications at the time of surgery

The immediate complications may be related to anaesthetic problems, for example, inability to intubate, anaphylaxis, or pulmonary oedema. Intra-operative damage to blood vessels leading to haemorrhage can occur and this can be particularly significant after prior radiotherapy. Direct damage to the bowel, ureter, or bladder is more common when the woman has had previous surgery. Failure of primary skin closure is sometimes seen in vulval surgery when wide excision or vulvectomy has been performed; a plastic surgical procedure is then needed.

The early post-operative period

In the early post-operative period (within two weeks of surgery), major and minor complications are quite common. These may be general complications seen in any surgical patient such as atelectasis, pneumonia, urinary retention and urinary tract infection, haematoma or wound infection either at the vaginal vault or in the abdominal incision, anaemia, ileus, wound dehiscence, thrombosis—deep vein, pelvic vein, and pulmonary embolus. A specific problem relating to radical surgery is bladder dysfunction which occurs in approximately 10 percent of patients due to the dissection around the pelvic nerves. This problem can occasionally continue for several months but recovery of bladder function is usually complete. Fistula (enterocutaneous, rectovaginal, vesicovaginal, or uretovaginal) occurs after about 1 percent of radical surgery and increases more than tenfold in frequency when the radical surgery is combined with radiotherapy. Further surgery is required to deal with this serious complication. Lymphocyst or lymphocele (a collection of lymphatic fluid in a pseudocyst) is sometimes seen after lymphadanectomy, in the pelvis or in the inguinal region. This gradually disappears.

Late complications

Late complications usually occur within one to three months of the operation. If a fistula develops as a late event, the usual cause is ischaemic damage. Treatment by diversion has already been discussed. Lympho-edema, unilateral or bilateral leg oedema, occurs after pelvic and inguinal lymphadenectomy in about 10–20 percent of cases. Treatment is difficult but bandaging and massage can provide relief in some cases. Strictures of any orifice (urethra, vagina, or stoma) or bowel arise due to scarring and internal structures may be related to adhesions. Hernias can either be internal when a bowel loop is caught between a band, causing obstruction, or protrude externally either through natural orifices, such as the vagina, or through the scar—incisional hernia. Surgery may be required. Sexual and psychological dysfunction affecting body image can be a cause of major morbidity and counselling is required (see Chapter 1, p. 7).

Early recurrence of tumour can occur. This may be the result of inadequate or incomplete surgery and is sometimes confused with granulation tissue at the vaginal vault or in the wound. Biopsy is important to differentiate between these two conditions. Death related to the surgery and its complications may occur at any time during the procedure and recovery, but is rare in modern oncology practice.

References

Holmesley, H. D., Bundy, B. N., Sedlis, A., and Adcock, L. (1986). Radiation therapy versus pelvic node resection for carcinoma of the vulva with positive groin nodes. *Obstetrics and Gynecology*, **68**, 733–40.

Piver, S., Rutledge, F., and Smith, J. P. (1974). Five classes of extended hysterectomy for women with cervical cancer. *Obstetrics and Gynecology*, **44**, 265–72.

Potter, M. E., Partridge, E. E., Hatch, K. D., Soong, S. J., Austin, J. M., and Shingleton, H. M. (1991). Primary surgical therapy of ovarian cancer: how much and when. *Gynecologic Oncology*, **40**, 195–200.

Shepherd, J. H., Ngan, H. Y. S., Neven, P., Fryatt, I., Woodhouse, C. R. J., and Hendry, W. F. (1994). Multivariate analysis of factors affecting survival in pelvic exenteration. *International Journal of Gynecological Cancer*, **4**, 361–70.

Young, R. C., Decker, D. G., Wharton, J. T., Piver, M. S., Sindelar, W. F.,Edwards, B. K., and Smith, J. P. (1983). Staging laparotomy in early ovarian cancer. *JAMA*, **250**, 3072–6.

Further reading

Colposcopy

Anderson, M., Jordan, J., Morse, A., and Sharp, F. (1992). *A text and atlas of integrated colposcopy*. Chapman and Hall, London.

9

Radiotherapy

Introduction

Radiotherapy is the therapeutic use of ionizing radiation. The discovery of X-rays and of radioactivity, by Wilhelm Roentgen and Henri Becquerel, respectively, occurred about 100 years ago. The potential value of these new discoveries as a means of treating a range of different conditions was appreciated very rapidly. Carcinoma of the cervix was one of the first tumours to be treated and radiotherapy has established itself as an effective therapeutic modality against a range of tumour types, including some of the common gynaecological cancers. Despite advances in other forms of anticancer therapies, it is likely that radiotherapy will continue to be a useful modality for the foreseeable future.

Radiation physics

Electromagnetic radiation

The electromagnetic spectrum (Fig. 9.1) describes the range of different electromagnetic radiations found in nature. The two types of electromagnetic radiation that are used in radiotherapy are X-rays and gamma rays. Both have short wavelengths ($<10^{-8}$ m), high frequencies, and carry high energies. Their physical properties are identical although their means of production vary.

X-rays are produced artificially by bombarding targets with high energy electrons. This process can occur in an X-ray tube or in a linear accelerator. During the resulting interactions between the atoms of the target and the electrons, X-rays are produced that have an energy dependent on the energy of the electrons. This energy is expressed in 'electron volts' and is usually in the mega electron volt (MeV) range.

Gamma rays are released by the nuclear decay of radioactive elements such as radium [^{226}Ra], cobalt [^{60}Co], caesium [^{137}Cs], and iridium [^{192}Ir]. Each radioactive isotope decays at a particular rate, or half-life, releasing gamma rays of different energies. Therefore, as rays of different energies penetrate tissues to different depths, the choice of radioisotope employed can be tailored to a particular clinical situation.

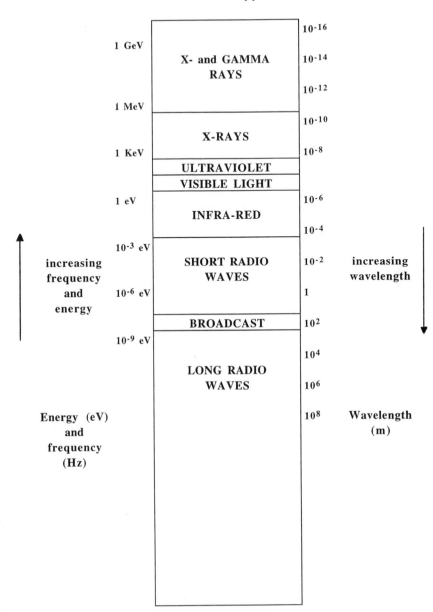

Fig. 9.1 The electromagnetic spectrum.

Particulate radiation

Particulate radiation consists of subatomic particles, including electrons, neutrons, protons, and alpha particles (nuclei of helium atoms). At present, the only commonly used type of particulate radiation is the high energy electron, which is generated by a linear accelerator, the most commonly used machine in radiotherapy. The beam of electrons is used directly from the machine rather than colliding with the target to produce X-rays. Electrons deliver their energy to tissue in a sparse manner and are called low linear energy transfer (LET) particles just as X- and gamma rays are low LET radiation.

Neutrons, protons, and alpha particles are densely ionizing and are produced by a cyclotron. They deliver large amounts of energy per unit length and are referred to as high LET particles. These have a greater relative effect on biological systems than X-rays, gamma rays, and electrons. In addition, high LET radiation is less dependent than low LET radiation on the presence of oxygen in the tissues for its cell-killing properties. Despite these apparently attractive characteristics, high LET radiation has failed to find a place in the routine treatment of common cancers because of technical difficulties in their production and adverse effects on normal tissues.

Radiobiology

Radiobiology is the study of the effects of radiation on living matter. Radiobiological effects in cells, tissues, and organs evolve through a series of phases, beginning with the physical absorption of energy into the system and ending with the biological effect, which can range from complete repair of damage to cell death. The principal means by which radiation interacts with biological systems is *directly* by means of inducing ionization and *indirectly* by generating free radicals as a result of radiation-induced lysis of water close to the DNA molecule. These interactions lead to damage in the deoxyribonucleic acid (DNA) in the cell nucleus, the critical target for ionizing radiation.

During radiotherapy normal tissues unavoidably receive some of the radiation dose. The effect of this absorbed dose in normal tissues is of major importance and imposes limits on the treatment that can be delivered safely. Normal tissue reactions are conventionally divided into *acute* and *late* reactions, depending on the cellular populations at risk and the timing of onset of the reactions. Acute reactions occur in rapidly proliferating tissues, such as bone marrow, skin, and the mucosae of the airway and gut, due to cell death in the stem cell population. Reactions like skin desquamation, radiation-induced diarrhoea, and mucosal ulceration belong to this category of radiation injury. They tend to be self-limiting and, if the dose has not been excessive, resolve rapidly without long-term sequelae. On the other hand, late reactions occur many weeks or months after the radiotherapy and are irreversible and often progressive. Their occurrence is due to vascular damage, probably at the level of the endothelial cell. Severe reactions such as bowel stenoses and fistulae, bladder fibrosis, and radiation-induced myelopathy may occur.

In general, it is the risk of late normal tissue damage that dominates clinical practice. Every course of radical radiotherapy involves balancing the chances of curing the disease against the risk of causing unacceptable late normal tissue damage. Figure 9.2 illustrates the essence of this dilemma and the relatively narrow therapeutic window within which curative treatment is given. In this hypothetical example, at a dose of 60 Gy very few tumours are cured but there are no adverse reactions. By increasing the dose to 65 Gy the cure rate is increased markedly to about 50 percent but this is achieved at the expense of 5 percent of the patients suffering a serious adverse

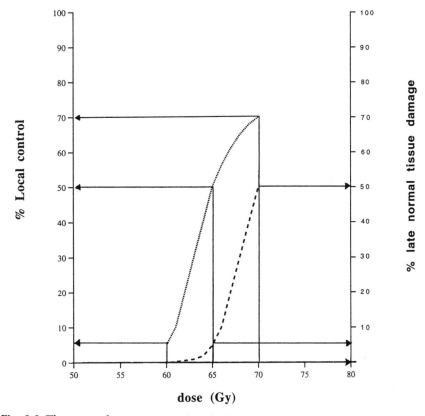

Fig. 9.2 The rates of tumour control and of severe complications with increasing radiation dose, a hypothetical example. Dotted line indicates tumour control; broken line indicates complication rate.

reaction. This equates to a complication-free cure rate of 45 percent. If attempts are made to increase the cure rate further by increasing the radiation dose to 70 Gy, 70 percent of patients are cured but 50 percent suffer complications, a complication-free survival of only 20 percent.

Although a detailed description of the science of radiobiology is beyond the scope of this text, a brief description of four of its central themes, often referred to as the four Rs of radiobiology, will highlight the important areas of interest. The four Rs are *repair*, *repopulation*, *re-oxygenation*, and *redistribution*.

Repair

The damage caused to the DNA of both normal and malignant cells by ionizing radiation can take a number of different forms. Single and double stranded breaks of the DNA are the most important phenomena and, in particular, double stranded breaks have been found to correlate with cell kill over a wide range of doses. However, once this damage has occurred it is not necessarily permanent as complex cellular mechanisms come into play to attempt to repair DNA damage and to restore the DNA code. It is thought that this repair is complete within six hours of irradiation. Although repair is a highly desirable property of normal cells, its occurrence in cancer cells will tend to reduce the tumour-killing ability of therapeutic radiation. The ability of normal and tumour cells to repair radiation-induced DNA damage varies and lies at the heart of the design of fraction-ated courses of radiotherapy.

Radiosensitivity parameters, *alpha* and *beta* are used in a linear quadratic model which mathematically describes the mechanisms involved in the ability of ionizing radiation to kill cells. *Alpha* measures the probability of causing lethal damage by a single event (non-reparable), whereas *beta* estimates the probability of cell death from two separate sublethal events (reparable damage that is not repaired). The *alpha:beta* ratio characterizes the way in which tissues and tumours respond to changes in fractionation or to dose rate in brachytherapy (p. 189). A low alpha:beta ratio (approx-imately 3Gy), indicating a high degree of sensitivity to changes in frac-tionation, characterizes those normal tissues which have a late response to the effects of radiation while a high alpha:beta ratio (approximately 10 Gy), indicating relative insensitivity to changes in fractionation, characterizes tumour cells and acutely reacting tissues.

The *therapeutic ratio* is the term used to describe the ratio between the cell kill in the tumour compared to that in the normal tissue. Changes in the pattern of fractionation alter the differential cell killing between tumours and late-responding normal tissues, in effect modifying the therapeutic ratio. Increasing the dose per fraction may be dangerous since this causes relatively more damage in normal tissues than in tumour and reduces the therapeutic ratio. On the other hand, reducing the dose per fraction may be advantageous as there will be differential sparing of normal tissues relative to tumour, increasing the therapeutic ratio. Balanced against this is the need to increase the total dose and number of fractions to achieve equal total tumour cell kill. If this requires undue prolongation of treatment the beneficial effects of fractionation may be lost by the occurrence of tumour cell repopulation and a decreased chance of cure. The alpha:beta ratios of the tumour and normal tissues can be used to calculate *biologically equivalent doses* for altered fractionation regimens.

With continuous brachytherapy, treatment given over many hours can be regarded as a large number of very small radiation fractions and repair occurs throughout the treatment. This gives rise to differential sparing of normal tissues while allowing high, curative doses to be delivered to the tumour. The situation is different in the case of high dose rate brachytherapy. This treatment has to be fractionated to allow repair of damage between the fractions which only last a few minutes. From first principles it would be predicted that a small number of large fractions of treatment at a high dose rate would cause unacceptable late tissue damage. However, with appropriate choice of fraction size and dose interval, safe and effective treatment has proved to be possible. The reason for this is that the physical and geometric factors, which apply to brachytherapy, ensure that the late responding normal tissues receive a lower dose per fraction than the tumour.

Repopulation

During a course of fractionated radiotherapy viable tumour cells continue to divide. As some cells are destroyed by a dose of radiation, new cells replace them. Some studies have suggested that after three weeks of fractionated radiotherapy viable clonogenic tumour cells are able to enter a phase of accelerated repopulation. Therefore, in order to eradicate a tumour completely, the radiotherapy must destroy not only all of the original tumour cells but also any formed by repopulation during the treatment period. This has led to the concept of 'wasted' radiation dose (i.e. some of the next fraction of radiotherapy is used up in killing cells born since the last fraction). It would be expected that prolongation of overall treatment times would be associated with an adverse effect on local control and patient survival. Clinical studies have confirmed this prediction for a number of different tumours, including carcinoma of the cervix. Changes in *conventional* fractionation regimens, when standard fractions are given once daily, usually five days a week, are being investigated. These include: *hyperfractionation* when an increased number of small fractions is given more than once daily within the same treatment time as conventional radiotherapy; and *accelerated hyperfractionation*, where the treatment is given more than once a day and in a shorter total period of time than conventional radiotherapy, but a gap in treatment is necessary to allow the acute radiation effects to resolve.

Re-oxygenation

Well-oxygenated cells are more susceptible to radiation-induced damage than hypoxic cells. This effect holds true for low LET radiation, such as X-rays, gamma rays, and electrons.

The well-oxygenated area around tumour blood vessels tends to contain healthy, dividing cells, whereas the areas distant from blood vessels often show areas of necrosis thought to be due to anoxic cell death. Radiotherapy is generally effective at killing the well-oxygenated cells around the blood vessels and those that have already died from anoxia no longer pose a problem. However, in the intervening area between well-oxygenated and anoxic cells are hypoxic cells that are able to remain viable only in a quiescent, non-cycling phase. There is considerable evidence that this population of cells is relatively radioresistant and is a major determinant of the outcome of therapy. Fractionation of radiotherapy provides a means of potentially circumventing this problem. It appears that between treatment fractions, as well-oxygenated cells are killed and cease to metabolize oxygen, oxygen is able to diffuse into hypoxic areas and reverse the relative radioresistance of previously hypoxic cells.

Redistribution

Cellular radiosensitivity varies at different phases of the cell cycle (see Fig. 10.2, p. 206). Cells in G_1, early S, and G_2/M phases are highly sensitive, whereas cells in late S phase are highly resistant to the effects of ionizing radiation. Fractionated courses of radiotherapy aim to exploit the tendency of tumour cells to redistribute into different phases of the cell cycle throughout the course of treatment. Therefore, it is hoped that cells in a relatively radioresistant phase at the time of one treatment fraction will be in a more sensitive phase at the time of the next fraction. This observation has led to attempts to accumulate cells in radiosensitive phases of the cell cycle. As yet, this has failed to result in clinical advances.

Units of measurement used in radiotherapy

The replacement of historical systems of measurement by the SI system of units (Système Internationale d'Unités) can lead to some confusion over nomenclature (Table 9.1). The SI unit of *absorbed dose* for external beam radiotherapy is the *gray* (Gy). This unit, which replaced the *rad*(r), is equivalent to the absorption of 1 joule of energy per kilogram of absorber. One gray is equivalent to 100 rads. *Exposure* to X-rays and gamma rays is

Table 9.1 Units of activity and dose

Quantity	Symbol	SI unit	Old unit	Relation
Activity	*A*	becquerel (Bq)	curie (Ci)	$1\ \text{Ci} = 3.7 \times 10^9\ \text{Bq}^*$
Dose	*D*	gray (Gy) = joules/kg	rad	$1\ \text{rad} = 10^{-2}\ \text{Gy}$
Kerma	*K*	gray (Gy) = joules/kg		
Exposure	*X*	coulomb (C)/kg	roentgen (R)	$1\ \text{R} = 2.58 \times 10^{-4}\ \text{C/kg}$

Note: this can also be expressed as 37 GBq (G = giga).

measured in *roentgen* (R) or coulombs/kg. The *activity* of radioactive sources is expressed in *becquerels* (Bq), which has replaced the *curie* (Ci) as the accepted unit, although the latter is still commonly used. In radiotherapy, activity measured in becquerels is usually in the mega- or giga-becquerel range as one becquerel is equal to one nuclear disintegration per second. In *radiation protection* the absorbed dose is described in terms of *sieverts* (Sv). This unit takes account of the relative biological effectiveness of the different types of radiation. For *brachytherapy* it has been recommended that measurement of the absorbed energy should be based on *kerma* (an acronym for kinetic energy released per unit mass). The unit of kerma (*K*) is the gray.

Radiotherapy techniques

Radiotherapy can be delivered in one of three ways: (1) teletherapy; (2) brachytherapy; or (3) by means of unsealed sources.

Teletherapy

This term refers to the use of treatment machines in which the source of radiation is distant from the patient. The treatment distance varies from 15-cm to more than 1 metre, but it is usually 100 cm. For this reason, this form of treatment is often referred to as 'external beam' radiotherapy. Production of radiation of teletherapy is based on the use of X-ray tubes, for energies less than 1 MeV, and linear accelerators (Fig. 9.3) or high activity radio-isotope sources for energies greater than 1 MeV.

Brachytherapy

Brachytherapy is the use of sealed radioactive sources contained within capsules or bonded covers which are placed in very close proximity to the treated tissue. This term embraces radiation sources which are placed on the surface of the tumour (moulds), in the lumen of a hollow viscus (intra-luminal), in a cavity (intracavitary), or within the substance of the tumour itself (interstitial). This treatment was initially developed when radium was

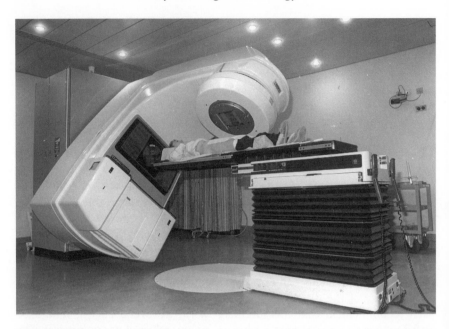

Fig. 9.3 A patient set up for treatment on a linear accelerator, the treatment head of which is capable of a 360 degree rotation around the treatment couch. The centre of the radiation beam is aligned with marks on the patient to ensure that the treatment is the same each day.

Table 9.2 Chief properties of radionuclides used frequently for brachytherapy (Trott 1987)

Radionuclide	Half-life	Principal energy (MeV)	Max. conc. available (GBq/mm^2)
Iridium-192 [^{192}Ir]	74.02 days	0.3–0.61	330
Cobalt-60 [^{60}Co]	5.27 years	1.17, 1.33	130
Caesium-137 [^{137}Cs]	30.00 years	0.66	1.2
Radium-226 [^{226}Ra]	1600 years	0.24–2.4	−0.05

the predominant radioisotope available. Nowadays, a number of radium substitutes, such as iridium and caesium, have been developed for clinical use (Table 9.2). Most gynaecological brachytherapy consists of temporary intracavitary placement of sources, although interstitial therapy may also be used. For each type of treatment there exists a detailed system for determining dosimetry, for example, the Manchester system for cancer of the cervix (Fig. 9.4) and the Paris system for interstitial implants.

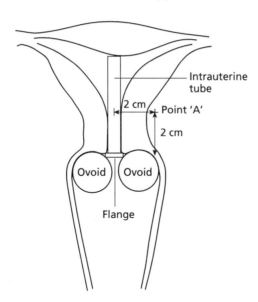

Fig. 9.4 The Manchester system for treatment of cancer of the cervix; Point 'A'.

Unsealed sources

Unsealed sources are radioactive materials which are not confined within a container and that come into direct contact with the patient. Unsealed sources are seldom used in the treatment of gynaecological cancers except for intraperitoneal therapy with ^{32}P-labelled colloids which have been given for early ovarian cancer.

External beam radiotherapy (teletherapy)

This technique allows therapeutic doses of radiation to be delivered to large volumes of tissue, such as those treated in patients with carcinoma of the cervix, in which the volume includes the tumour itself, the parametria and the loco-regional lymph nodes.

Dose prescription

The radiation dose prescription for external beam radiotherapy includes the *total dose*, the *total number of treatment fractions*, the *total treatment time*, the *dose per fraction*, the *point at which the dose is prescribed*, and the *energy of the radiation*. For example, a prescription for external beam radiotherapy to the pelvis could be 45 Gy in 25 fractions given 5 times per week over 5 weeks at 1.8 Gy per fraction delivered to the centre point of the planning treatment volume (see below) using 8 MeV X-rays.

Treatment volumes

During the process of planning radiotherapy, a number of different volumes of tissue need to be considered (Fig. 9.5). The *gross tumour volume* (GTV) describes the macroscopic extent of the tumour that is palpable, visible, or demonstrable on imaging. The GTV includes the primary tumour and gross loco-regional extension (e.g. to local lymph nodes) and represents the stage of disease. It cannot be defined if the tumour has been removed. The *clinical tumour volume* (CTV) encompasses the GTV with an additional margin to take account of likely routes of spread. For instance loco-regional lymph nodes suspected of containing subclinical microdeposits of disease will be included in the CTV. It is this volume of tissue which is judged to be at risk and which needs to be sterilized. To ensure that all the tissues included in the CTV receive the prescribed dose of radiation a margin is added to take account of day-to-day variation in treatment set-up and movement during treatment. This *planning target volume* (PTV) is used to plan the dose distribution to the CTV. The actual *treatment volume* is the volume of tissue enclosed by an isodose surface (a line joining two or more points receiving the same dose of radiation), the value of which is the minimum target absorbed dose (usually 95 percent of the prescribed dose). This volume is usually slightly larger than the PTV and depends to some extent on the treatment technique used.

Ideally, dose should *only* be delivered to areas containing macroscopic or microscopic disease. However, this is not possible and a much larger volume of tissue will receive some radiation either from entry or exit of the beams or

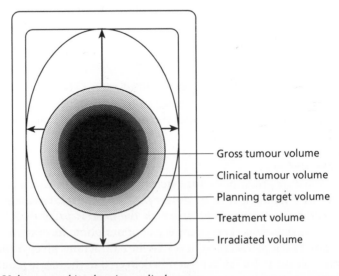

Gross tumour volume

Clinical tumour volume

Planning target volume

Treatment volume

Irradiated volume

Fig. 9.5 Volumes used in planning radiotherapy.

from scatter within the body. This *irradiated volume* is the volume of tissue which absorbs a dose deemed to be significant in terms of the tissues contained therein.

Treatment planning

The aim of radiotherapy planning is to ensure delivery of a homogenous dose to the clinical tumour volume whilst minimizing the dose to surrounding normal tissues. The volume of tissue to be treated is measured in three dimensions superior-inferior, anterior-posterior, and right to left laterally. Accurate localization of the volume to be treated is essential and is achieved by collating information from clinical examination, surgico-pathological findings, and radiological investigations (plain radiographs, ultrasound, CT, and MRI scanning). The dose of radiation that will be tolerated by normal tissues within the irradiated volume must be known. Particular attention must be given to critical normal organs such as the spinal cord, kidneys and liver, as these organs will not tolerate high doses of radiation.

The size of the treatment volume and the overall dose will be influenced by the age and general condition of the patient. For example, arteriosclerosis and bowel disease, such as diverticular disease, both reduce the bowel's tolerance of radiation. Small bowel tolerates only low doses of radiation but, during a fractionated course of radiotherapy, its mobility enables it to move in and out of the radiation field, thus reducing the total dose that it receives. However, in patients who have undergone prior surgery the bowel may be fixed by adhesions and may be more susceptible to radiation damage. Care must be taken to avoid excessive doses of radiation to the rectum and pelvic colon, which will inevitably form part of the treatment volume for pelvic tumours.

Planning procedure

The treatment is simulated by positioning the patient on a *simulator*, a mobile couch beneath a fluoroscopy unit producing diagnostic X-rays, which generates an image on a television screen (Fig. 9.6). Localization of the *planning target volume* (PTV) is achieved and the surface markings of this volume are projected on to the patient's skin using a beam of light defining the margins of the radiotherapy field. A radiographic film is taken as a permanent record and the field edges are drawn on the patient's skin with a semi-permanent marker pen. Small tattoo marks are often made on the skin surface to define points which provide important landmarks for aligning the patient correctly on the treatment machines each day. A tracing of the body *contour* is made in the form of a transverse slice at the level of the volume centre, either manually by outlining the area with pliable wire and transferring the shape to paper or by using a CT planning computer. On

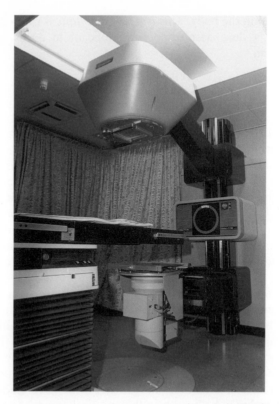

Fig. 9.6 A simulator for treatment planning of patients for radiotherapy using light beams in place of X-rays.

this contour the planning target volume will be drawn using a CT planning computer (Fig. 9.7a).

For the tumour to receive a therapeutic radiation dose without overdosing the overlying skin or other normal tissues, several fields arranged at different angles with different entry points are used. A planning computer calculates the field sizes, the angular arrangement of the fields, and the relative dose distribution between the fields that is required to deliver a homogenous dose to the tumour. The computerized plan of the final radiation dose delivered by means of a three field plan to the pelvis in a patient with carcinoma of the cervix is shown in Figs. 9.7b,c,d. The most commonly used field arrangements employ between two and four fields, but techniques in which a radiation source rotates around the centre of the treatment volume are occasionally used. Newer linear accelerators have the ability to produce irregularly shaped fields by the use of multi-leaf collimators. This allows accurate shielding of critical normal structures with the potential benefits of

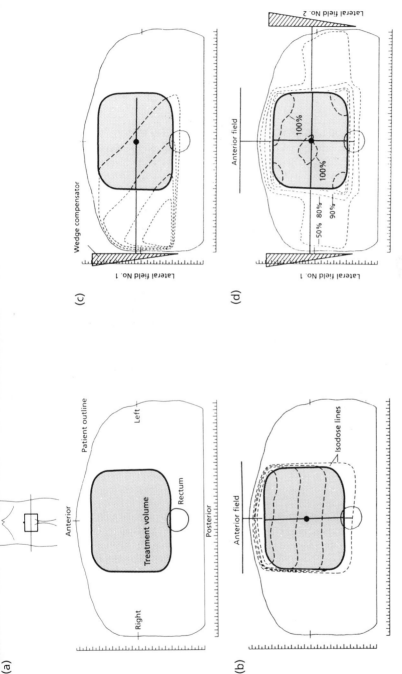

Fig. 9.7 A computerized plan for a patient with carcinoma of the cervix. The four diagrams (a, b, c, d) show how a planning computer can build up the dose distribution that best fits the treatment volume drawn on to the patient outline by the radiotherapist. The 'isodose' lines join all points receiving the same dose. The dose falls with increasing distance from the source of radiation and so isodose lines may either be given as an actual dose value or as a percentage figure of the maximum dose in the tissues (e.g. 90 percent). In this case, to give an even dose to the treatment volume, the final plan uses an anterior and two lateral fields.

reducing normal tissue toxicity and allowing escalation of the dose delivered to the tumour. This is particularly useful for treating small volumes in the pelvis or para-aortic nodes.

Tissue compensators may be used to increase the homogeneity of dose distribution in the treatment volume. For instance, wedge-shaped compensators are generally used in the lateral fields of a three-field treatment arrangement for cancer of the cervix and endometrium. Alternatively, thick lead blocks can be interposed in the treatment beam to shield critical normal structures from doses which would exceed their radiation tolerance (Fig. 9.8).

Implementation of the treatment plan

Treatment is given.in specially constructed treatment rooms, or bunkers, which comply with radiation protection guidelines. The patient lies on a treatment couch in the same position as defined on the simulator couch. The field size, machine angle, and the presence or absence of lead blocks and tissue compensators are set for each treatment field. Radiographers, who treat the patient, use a control console outside to set the radiation dose and to start and stop the machine. The treatment time for each field is usually less than one minute and may only be a few seconds. The patient is alone in the treatment room whilst the radiation beam is on but is supervised throughout by means of closed-circuit television. Voice contact by a two-way microphone is usually possible.

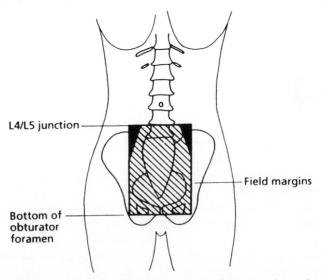

L4/L5 junction

Field margins

Bottom of
obturator
foramen

Fig. 9.8 The anterior field used for irradiation of the planning volume showing the position of lead blocks to shield the small bowel in the upper corners of the volume.

On each treatment machine a range of technical checks is made each day before treatment begins. In addition, machines are serviced regularly to ensure accuracy of dose delivery. During patient treatment, a number of independent systems are in operation to ensure that accurate treatment is delivered.

Gynaecological intracavitary brachytherapy

The chief advantage of this form of treatment, in which a radioactive source is placed within a hollow organ, such as the uterus and vagina, is that it allows a very high dose to be delivered to a small volume of tissue immediately adjacent to the radioactive sources. Beyond this there is a very rapid fall-off of dose due to the effect of the inverse square law. Until the recent development of high dose rate systems using microsources, the main application of brachytherapy was in treating gynaecological malignancies.

Clinical uses

The main use for intravcavitary brachytherapy is in the treatment of cancer of the cervix but it may also be used in the management of cancers of the endometrium and of the vagina. Details are given in the chapters covering these tumours. Brachytherapy as sole treatment is only applicable to very early tumours and usually treatment consists of a combination of external radiotherapy to treat the clinical treatment volume and brachytherapy to give a high dose of radiotherapy to a small volume at the site of the tumour.

History

In the 1920s, work at the Radiumhemmet in Stockholm and at the Curie Foundation in Paris resulted in the development of the 'Stockholm system' and the 'Paris system' for the treatment of uterine cancer using intracavitary radium sources in the uterus and vagina. The Stockholm system was based on using relatively large amounts of radium and the treatment was fractionated into two or three equal parts each lasting 20–24 hours, two or three weeks apart. In contrast, the Paris system used less radium and irradiation was continuous over a period of 6–8 days.

The Manchester system, which uses an intrauterine tube and 2 vaginal applicators, one in each vaginal fornix, was designed in the 1930s and was based on the concept that the limiting dose to normal tissue should be measured in the area where the ureter crossed the uterine artery, the 'paracervical triangle'. *Point A*, a point used to assess dose in this triangle, was defined as 2 cm lateral to the uterine canal and 2 cm above the mucous membrane of the lateral vaginal fornix, in the plane of the uterus. *In practice*, this point is measured from X-rays as 2 cm lateral to the radioactive uterine source and 2 cm superior to its inferior surface (see Fig. 9.4).

Point B, a further reference point, was defined as 5 cm from the midline and 2 cm superior to the lateral vaginal fornix. This point gives the dose in the vicinity of the pelvic wall, near the obturator node and is also an indication of the lateral spread of the effective dose.

The uterine tubes were of 3 different active lengths, short (2 cm), medium (4 cm), and long (6 cm), and the vaginal applicators—ovoids, which were ellipsoid to correspond to the isodose curves, were designed as small (2 cm), medium (2.5 cm), and large (3 cm) in diameter. The activity and arrangement of the sources was made to ensure that the dose rate at point A was 0.54 Gy/hour and a total dose of 75–80 Gy was given in 2 fractions over 6 days, whatever combination of sources was used. The dose at point B was 25–30 percent of the dose at point A. The Manchester system remains the basis for intracavitary therapy in the UK.

The Fletcher–Houston system used in the USA, and designed in the 1950s, is a development of the Manchester system which uses cylindrical colpostats in place of ovoids, which have separate handles that can be locked together at a scissor joint. This allows the vagina to be distended laterally with a resultant increase in dose to the paracervical and parametrial tissues. The vaginal applicators contain tungsten shields which modify the dose to the rectum and bladder.

After-loading

Most radiotherapy centres have replaced the direct insertion of radioactive sources into a patient with an after-loading system. These can be manually or remotely controlled and they can deliver low, medium, or high dose rates (Table 3.6, p. 67). These systems allow time to be taken over the positioning of applicators without hazard to the operator. Only after the accuracy of their placement has been verified by X-ray films are the radioactive sources inserted. Although manual systems are comparatively cheap, they do not avoid all irradiation to staff. The complexity of remote systems means that they are expensive to run and require more staff with the necessary expertise. However, they not only protect all personnel involved with the procedure but, because they are faster than traditional methods, they allow more patients to be treated in a given time, making them cost-effective for a large patient load. In addition, the very short treatment times possible with high dose rate brachytherapy ensure geometrical stability of the applicators throughout treatment.

Manual after-loading techniques (low dose rate)

In manual after-loading systems the radioactive sources, in their source trains, are loaded by hand into the applicators after the patient has returned to the ward. This eliminates exposure to radiation of theatre staff but does not allow complete staff protection. The most commonly used manual after-loading system is that manufactured by Amersham International, which reproduces the Manchester technique and uses sources of caesium [^{137}Cs]. It consists of disposable, flexible plastic tubes with the ovoids, spacers, and washers being made of high impact polystyrene. The applicators, which are impregnated with barium so that they can easily be seen on X-ray, separate into sections which can be held together by a polystyrene disc through which the sections pass (Fig. 9.9).

Remote-controlled after-loading (low and medium dose rate)

Remote after-loading systems allow complete staff protection. The source can be in the form of a single capsule or in a series of capsules. Source transfer from the safe to the patient can be in a flexible spring attached to a cable, or can be pneumatic. There are several systems commercially available including the Curietron and the Selectron. The Curietron makes use of flexible source trains, which consist of ^{137}Cs sealed sources (1.5 mm diameter and 3.5 mm long) and spacers loaded into a stainless steel spring and closed at one end. The end distal to the source train is sealed with a hook which identifies the train and provides a means of connection to one of the drive cables. The sources are returned to the safe when the treatment is completed. Up to four source trains, each with their own configuration, can be used at any one time and different configurations are made at the time of manufacture.

In the Selectron machine, the caesium sources are in the form of 2.5 mm diameter spherical pellets. The source trains can be made up of a combination of 48 sources and spacers, and the number and position of the active sources in each source train can be independently programmed using

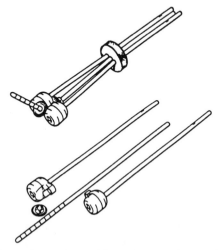

Fig. 9.9 The Amersham plastic disposable applicator after-loading system.

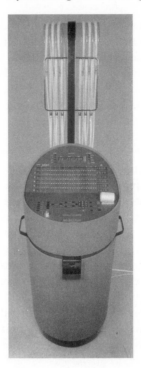

Fig. 9.10 The Selectron 'low' dose rate after-loading machine. Radioactive caesium-137 pellets are delivered into the applicators in the patient by a pneumatic system. Six applicators can be used at the same time, thus enabling two patients to be treated simultaneously.

a computer system. The sources are sorted from the spacers magnetically and are transferred pneumatically into the patient via flexible tubing that fits on to the end of stainless steel applicators (Fig. 9.10).

Classically, the dose rate to point A with the Manchester system is 0.54 Gy/hour but with remote after-loading systems, such as the Curietron or Selectron, the dose rate of brachytherapy can be increased. Caesium pellets can be produced with an activity allowing a dose rate of between 1.5 and 2 Gy/hour. This allows for shorter treatment times. For example, when a patient with stage Ib cervical cancer is treated by intracavitary therapy alone, using standard dose rate to give 70–80 Gy to point A, treatment takes approximately 6 days, with 2 fractions being given over 3 days each separated by a 4-day gap. By increasing the dose rate by a factor of three, the treatment time for each of the 2 fractions, is reduced to 1 day. This is more cost-effective. Many systems now use sources that deliver a higher than standard dose rate whilst remaining in the low dose range as defined by the International Committee on Radiological Units (ICRU 1984) (Table 3.6,

p. 67). The increased dose rate necessitates a reduction in *total dose* to give an equivalent biological dose to the standard system in order to prevent severe radiation complications (see p. 194).

Remote-controlled after-loading (high dose rate)

High dose rate after-loading, in which treatment times are measured in *minutes* rather than hours, requires radioisotopes of very high specific activity. ^{60}Co and ^{192}Ir are the only radioactive isotopes with a very high specific activity that satisfy the requirements that an after-loading source emits radiation of a suitable energy, is solid, has solid decay products, is capable of being worked, and is non-soluble. Cobalt has the advantage that it has a half-life of over 5 years rather than 74 days for iridium and, therefore, needs replacement only every 3–6 years compared to every 3–4 months. However, gamma rays from ^{192}Ir are much less penetrating than those from ^{60}Co and require less shielding in storage (Table 9.2).

Very high activity cobalt sources were first used for high dose-rate brachytherapy in the late 1960s, with the Cathetron machine. The development in the 1980s of very small iridium sources of less than 1 mm diameter enabled the manufacture of applicators with diameters of less than 4 mm (compared to the 6 mm needed for cobalt or caesium) thus increasing the ease of insertion and the uses for brachytherapy at both gynaecological and other sites. A set of remote after-loading applicators for the microSelectron is shown in Fig. 9.11.

Two machines, the microSelectron HDR (Fig. 9.12) and the Gammamed 12, are the main high dose rate machines in use in the UK. Both use a cable-driven, small, high activity ^{192}Ir source to give brachytherapy. Source position can be altered in a stepwise fashion with variable dwell times to give different distributions of radiation. Dose rates are in excess of 1 Gy/min to point A.

As explained earlier, normal tissues undergo some repair of radiation damage during continuous low dose rate intracavitary treatment, but the time taken for a high dose rate treatment is too short for this to occur.

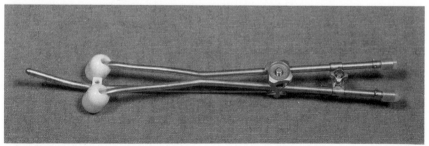

Fig. 9.11 A set of remote after-loading applicators with a central intrauterine tube and two lateral vaginal applicators.

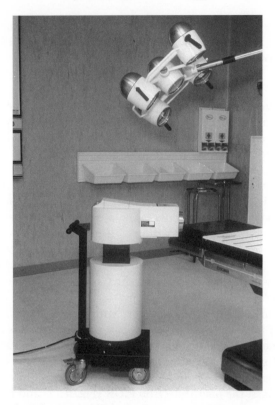

Fig. 9.12 The microSelectron HDR 'high' dose rate machine.

Therefore, high dose rate treatments have to be divided into several fractions, in the same way as external radiotherapy, to allow this repair to take place, otherwise the damage to normal tissues would be unacceptable. For the same reason it is also necessary to reduce the total dose of radiation given with high dose rate therapy compared to that given with continuous low dose rate systems. This reduction in dosage has not been found to make high dose rate treatment less effective in curing cervical cancer (p. 196).

Procedure for intracavitary therapy

A general anaesthetic is usually needed to allow insertion of the uterine tube through the cervix. A prostaglandin pessary inserted into the vault of the vagina, 2–3 hours before the procedure, makes cervical dilatation much easier, as this can be difficult following destruction of cervical tissues by tumour and radiation (Harrington *et al.* 1994). Following dilatation of the cervix the length of the uterine cavity is measured to allow the correct uterine tube to be selected. The width of the vaginal vault is determined and the vaginal ovoids chosen. The bladder is catherized with a Foley catheter. The balloon is filled with 7 ml radiopaque fluid and pulled down on to the bladder base. The dose received by the bladder base can subsequently be calculated as the balloon is visible on the radiograph. After the uterine tube has been inserted, the vaginal ovoids are positioned, one in each lateral fornix, and the vagina is packed with gauze. This packing may be used to displace the vault applicators forward, reducing the dose of radiation received by the rectum and also ensuring stability of the set-up during treatment. Alternatively, the rectal dose can be reduced by placing special spacers in the vagina that are designed to push the rectum away from the sources. The dose delivered to the tumour and to the surrounding organs, rectum and bladder, are calculated from anterior-posterior and lateral radiographs, using the appropriate isodose charts available for each brachy-therapy system. Alternatively, with manual after-loading systems, direct measurement of the rectal dose can be made, using a rectal dosimeter.

Intracavitary dose prescription and recording

For intracavitary brachytherapy the dose prescription varies according to the treatment applicators used, which will depend on the disease being treated. Information should be available on the *total dose*, the *point at which the dose is prescribed*, the *number of insertions*, the *interval between insertions*, the *dose rate*, and the *applicators used*. With Manchester-type applicators comprising an intrauterine tube and two vaginal ovoids, a prescription for intracavitary brachytherapy to the cervix is, as described previously, prescribed to point A. For example, using a 6 cm intrauterine tube with two medium vaginal ovoids following external radiotherapy, this prescription dose could be 16.5 Gy to point A, in 3 insertions performed once per week, using the high dose rate microSelectron, delivering at a dose rate of 1 Gy per minute.

For accurate dosimetry, information on the geometrical relation of the applicators to each other and to the patient is needed. This is obtained by the anterior-posterior radiographs, mentioned above, which show the applicators in relation to the patient. Also, for low dose rate systems the exact *activity* and *distribution* of sources within the applicators or, for high dose rate systems, the exact *dwell positions* and *dwell times* of the source must be recorded.

In many cases the intracavitary treatment will be part of a combined approach with external radiotherapy. The external beam dose must then be expressed separately.

ICRU intracavitary therapy dose recording

The International Commission on Radiological Units (ICRU 1985) have issued specific recommendations for reporting intracavitary therapy in gynaecology. Fundamental to these requirements is the need for dosimetry in orthogonal planes. Most computer treatment planning systems use data obtained from X-rays taken at different angles.

Dose and volume specification.   The dose gradient near to the radioactive sources is too high for specifying doses at target points and the ICRU recommend the use of a *dose volume specification* which should be used with the *total reference air kerma* for a patient's treatment. A kerma, as previously described is equivalent to a gray. The *total reference air kerma* is the sum of the products of the *reference air kerma* and the duration of the application for each source; the reference air kerma being the kerma rate to air measured at a distance of 1 metre from the source. In addition to these measurements, the absorbed dose at reference points related to organs at risk or to bony structures is recommended as well as details of the time-dose pattern.

Description of the reference volume.   The tissue volume encompassed by a reference isodose should be specified. For this one needs the *reference dose level*, the *description of the reference volume*, and the recording of *dose at various reference points.*

For classical low dose rate therapy an absorbed dose level of 60 Gy is accepted as the appropriate reference level from all insertions. When intracavitary therapy is combined with external beam therapy, the isodose level to be considered is the difference between 60 Gy and the dose delivered at the same location by external beam therapy. When the intracavitary therapy is medium or high dose rate, the reference isodose level is that considered to be equivalent to 60 Gy.

The reference volume from the combination of Manchester-type uterine and vaginal sources is 'pear-shaped', with its longest axis coincident with the uterine source (Fig. 9.13). The reference volume is determined from the

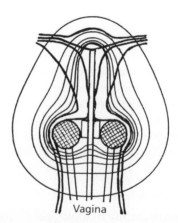

Fig. 9.13 The 'pear-shaped' isodose pattern achieved in the anterior–posterior plane by the Manchester system.

radiographs of the insertion and is defined in three dimensions height, width, and thickness, all expressed in centimetres. The height is the maximum dimension along the plane of the intrauterine source. The width is the maximum dimension perpendicular to the uterine source in the lateral plane and the thickness is the maximum dimension perpendicular to the intrauterine source measured in the anterior-posterior plane (Fig. 9.14).

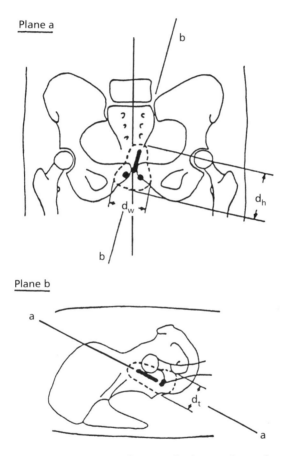

Fig. 9.14 ICRU Report 38 (1985). Specification of reference dose volume. Geometry for measurement of the 'pear-shaped' 60 Gy isodose surface (broken line) in a typical treatment of cervix carcinoma using one rod-shaped uterine applicator and 2 vaginal applicators. *Plane a* is the 'oblique' frontal plane that contains the intrauterine device. *Plane b* is the 'oblique' sagittal plane that contains the intrauterine device. The height (d_h) and the width (d_w) of the reference volume are measured in *plane a* as the maximal sizes parallel and perpendicular to the uterine applicator, respectively. The thickness (d_t) is measured in *plane b* as the maximal size perpendicular to the uterine applicator.

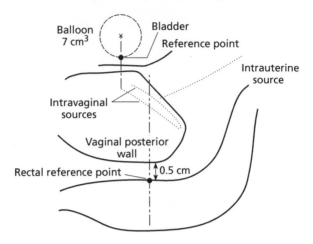

Fig. 9.15 ICRU Report 38 (1985). Measurement of doses to bladder and rectum.

Recommended reference points include those relatively close to the sources but related to organs at risk, the bladder and rectum, and those more distant, related to bony structures. The *bladder reference point* is obtained from a lateral X-ray, by drawing a line through the centre of the balloon of a Foley catheter, containing 7 cm^3 of radiopaque fluid, and pulled down to lie in contact with the urethra. The reference point is taken on this line at the posterior surface of the balloon. On the anterior-posterior radiograph, the reference point is taken as the centre of the balloon (Fig. 9.15).

The *rectal reference point* on the lateral radiograph is obtained by drawing an anterior-posterior line from the lower end of the intrauterine source (or from the middle of the intravaginal sources). The point is located on this line 5 mm behind the posterior vaginal wall which is visualized by the radiopaque gauze used for packing or the back of the vaginal applicators. On the anterior-posterior radiograph this reference point is at the lower end of the intrauterine source or at the middle of the vaginal sources (Fig. 9.15).

Reference points to bony structures are useful for estimating the dose received by pelvic nodes from intracavitary irradiation. This is particularly useful when intracavitary therapy is combined with external beam therapy (Fig. 9.16).

Modification of dose prescription for medium dose rate brachytherapy

With modern remote after-loading machines dose rates are commonly between 1.5 and 1.8 Gy per hour. Whilst this is still low dose rate therapy,

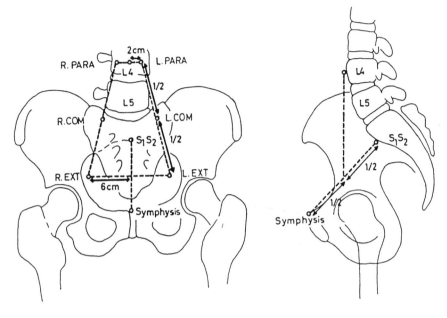

Fig. 9.16 ICRU Report 38 (1985). Specification of reference points related to bony structures (Right and left para-aortic, common iliac and external iliac node groups).

according to the ICRU definition (Table 3.6, p. 87), clinical experience has shown that a dose reduction is needed to maintain an isoeffect with the standard dose rate of 0.54 Gy/hour, as given with the classical Manchester system. Studies in Manchester compared 75 Gy to point A from 2 radium insertions, each lasting 70 hours, with varying doses from caesium given at a dose rate of 1.4–1.8 Gy/hour, depending on the decay of the caesium-137. The study showed that a total dose of 60 Gy compared to higher doses of up to 75 Gy, gave a shorter disease-free survival but that high doses were associated with more severe mordibity (Hunter 1995).

In those patients treated with a combination of external radiotherapy and brachytherapy, the results in terms of survival, primary disease control and complications were the same in those patients treated with radium and those treated with caesium, with either a 9 percent or 17 percent dose reduction. Therefore, a dose reduction of about 10 percent should suffice. This reduction of 10 percent in total dose is also suggested by Brenner and Hall (1991). For those patients treated with *intracavitary therapy alone*, the Manchester studies (Hunter 1995) suggested that a larger dose correction factor, in the range of 12.5–20 percent, was needed to avoid undue morbidity.

Modification of dose prescription for high dose rate brachytherapy

With high dose rates, comparisons with low dose rates are difficult as few comparative studies have been carried out but, overall, they suggest similar results in regard to survival, local control, and complication rates (Fu and Phillips 1990; Khoury *et al.* 1991).

The ideal time/dose/fractionation scheme and its integration with external radiotherapy has yet to be developed but one randomized study, that of Sharma *et al.* (1991), illustrates a successful regimen and gives some indication of how much the standard low dose rate (LDR) dose should be reduced when using high dose rate (HDR) therapy. Over 400 patients participated in the study and all had pelvic radiotherapy, receiving 45 Gy in 20 fractions over 4 weeks. Half the patients then received LDR brachytherapy giving 35 Gy to point A in one fraction and the others having HDR therapy receiving 17 Gy, 18 Gy, or 19 Gy to point A in 2 fractions. Apart from a higher incidence of acute vaginal hyperaemia in the HDR group, there was no significant difference in the complication rate (Table 9.3). The recurrence rate in the group that received 17 Gy to point A was higher than for any of the other groups but the numbers were small (Table 9.4).

In general, it has been found that to avoid an unacceptable normal tissue complication rate or local recurrence rate, the dose given at high dose rate

Table 9.3 Complication rate of low dose rate (LDR) and high dose rate (HDR) regimens (Sharma *et al.* 1991)

Complication	Low dose rate (220 patients)	High dose rate (203 patients)
Urinary bladder		
Frequency	0	3
Haematuria	4	3
Vagina		
Hyperaemia	0	34
Adhesions/stenosis	3	6
Telangiectasia	2	5
Rectosigmoid		
Grade 1*	35	18
Grade 2*	3	0
Grade 3*	4	0

* ECOG toxicity criteria:
Grade 1 Transient diarrhoea lasting 2 days or less.
Grade 2 Tolerable diarrhoea lasting more than 2 days.
Grade 3 Intolerable diarrhoea requiring therapy.

Table 9.4 Local failure related to intracavitary dose: low dose rate (LDR) vs high dose rate (HDR) (Sharma *et al.* 1991)

LDR/HDR	No. of patients	Residual disease	Local recurrence	Total no. of local failures	% of local failures
LDR (35 Gy)	220	22	9	31	14
HDR (17 Gy/2 f*)	27	6	3	9	33
HDR (18 Gy/2 f)	35	3	1	4	11
HDR (19 Gy/2 f)	141	14	6	20	14

*f, fractions.

should be in the region of 55–70 percent of the dose given at low dose rate, the fraction size should not exceed 8–10 Gy and treatments should be between one and three times per week.

Interstitial brachytherapy

In general, external radiotherapy with electrons has largely replaced the need for interstitial brachytherapy as this allows an even dose distribution with a limited depth, depending on the energy of the electrons used. For example, 10 MeV electrons will treat to a depth of 2.5 cm with little radiation beyond, thus limiting the irradiated volume. However, in some areas, such as the lower vagina and the parametria, interstitial brachytherapy is more suitable than electrons for treatment.

Radium needles have been replaced by other isotopes, usually iridium –192, used in wires or seeds that can be manually after-loaded into hollow tubes or inserted using remote after-loading with the microSelectron. After-loading allows the correct geometrical arrangement of tubes, which can be a lengthy procedure that would be hazardous if active sources were used. When implanting lesions of the lower vagina, a particular problem arises because the tubes, although parallel when inserted with the patient in the lithotomy position, tend to move when the legs are lowered at the end of the procedure. The introital end of the applicators crowd together, while the cranial ends splay apart. A perspex template sewn to the perineum can be used to ensure that the applicators remain parallel and at a fixed distance from one another. This ensures a good dose distribution in the implanted volume without the occurrence of 'hot' or 'cold' spots. Although the appearance of the template is rather forbidding, with careful nursing it is remarkably well tolerated (Fig. 5.4, p. 117).

Dose prescription

Because of the very rapid fall-off in dose rate as distance from a radiation source increases it is inevitable that, if sources are placed directly in tissues, there will be a very inhomogenous dose distribution with 'hot-spots' around the sources. However, both the Manchester and Paris systems of dosimetry ignore the very high dose rate areas within 5 mm of the implanted sources and try to ensure, by accurate and regular placement of sources, that the dose rate in the rest of the implanted volume is relatively homogenous. The technique of implanting the sources is specialized and the calculation of dose rate is difficult, usually requiring a computer. If a volume were to be implanted for the treatment of a tumour by interstitial therapy alone the dose prescribed should be in the region of 60 Gy to the volume over six days. In addition to the dose, the isotope and method of dosimetry should be recorded.

Unsealed radioisotope therapy

Radiotherapy for small volume disease in the peritoneal and pleural spaces can be delivered using a radioisotope solution. Early stage ovarian cancers have been treated using intraperitoneal radioactive phosphorus linked to colloids, the latter to prevent a too rapid absorption. This gives a high radiation dose but only to a depth of 4–6 mm, limiting therapy to small superficial deposits. There is no evidence that this improves survival in patients with these early tumours. Radioactive labelled monoclonal antibodies have been used in the same way in an attempt to target the treatment to tumour cells and early results show that this therapy extends survival in patients who are in complete remission after adjuvant chemotherapy.

Dose prescription

In situations where unsealed sources are used accurate specification of radiation dose is very difficult. In general, the doses administered are expressed either in terms of total activity, activity per kg, or activity per unit of body surface area [e.g. 1 GBq (27 mCi)/m^2]. Safe doses are derived from the results of phase I dose-finding studies.

Radiation protection

In 1985, the Ionizing Radiation Regulations were passed as a statutory, legally binding set of rules issued under the authority of the Health and Safety Executive. The aim of these regulations is to ensure adequate protection of hospital staff, patients, visitors, and other members of the general public from the adverse effects of unwanted exposure to ionizing radiation. The general approach to this problem is to restrict the use of ionizing radiation to justifiable situations, to ensure that radiation exposure is as low as is reasonably achievable (ALARA), and to lay down legal dose limits. These limits are specified in terms of dose equivalents, which are derived from the absorbed dose (in Gy), multiplied by a 'quality factor', which takes account of the relative biological effectiveness (RBE) of different types of radiation. The quality factor for X-rays, gamma rays, and electrons is 1.0, whereas that for fast neutrons and alpha particles is 10–20. Therefore, the dose equivalent from 1 Gy of X-ray irradiation is 1 sievert (Sv), whereas that from 1 Gy of fast neutrons is 10–20 Sv. Strict legal dose limits are in operation, which differ between different members of staff and the general public. In addition, the limits for whole-body irradiation are lower than those for parts of the body, such as the hands of staff recognized as radiation workers.

When working with or near radioactive sources, three simple practical guidelines can be used to reduce the dose received:

1. Exposure time should be minimized since the absorbed dose is cumulative.

2. Distance from the source should be maximized whenever possible. The dose rate of a radiation source is inversely proportional to the square of the distance from it. Therefore, by doubling one's distance from the source, the dose is reduced to one-quarter.

3. Attenuating or shielding materials should be used whenever possible. High density materials, such as lead and concrete, reduce dose levels very effectively. This factor is employed in constructing the bunkers that house linear accelerators, the walls of which may be more than 2 metres thick.

Radiation damage to normal tissues

Treatment regimens are designed with the assumption that all patients have a similar sensitivity to therapeutic radiation but, as discussed earlier, there is a large difference in normal tissue sensitivity between patients. At the present time, a rapid and accurate assay to assess radiosensitivity is not available and only crude criteria can be used, with the exception of those very rare patients with conditions such as telengectasia-ataxia who are identifiable as being highly radiation-sensitive. These crude criteria include those patients who are very fair, have rheumatoid arthritis, diabetic vascular changes, and, when the pelvis is being treated, those patients with inflammatory bowel disease such as Crohn's disease and ulcerative colitis.

Regimens are designed to give maximum cure rates with minimum morbidity. The radiation tolerance of normal tissue will depend on:

(a) the volume being irradiated;

(b) the total dose and dose rate; and

(c) the size of the fractions.

Some organs are more susceptible than others to radiation damage, such as the spinal cord, kidneys, and small bowel. The dose tolerance for such organs needs to be known when planning radiotherapy, if irreversible damage is to be avoided. A way of expressing this dose tolerance is by the dose that gives a given complication in 5 percent of patients in 5 years: the *tolerance dose* (TD)5/5. The TD5/5 for late complications with fractionated radiation is 65 Gy for bladder, 65 Gy for rectum, 50 Gy for bowel, and 50 Gy for spinal cord (Orner *et al.* 1996). Usually, doses to the rectum and bladder are kept at a maximum of this TD5/5 dose of 65 Gy delivered to a single maximum reference point.

Normal tissue reactions occur both early and late. Early tissue reactions take place during or immediately after a course of radiotherapy but recovery is usually rapid. Late reactions occur from about one year onwards, are permanent, and are usually slowly progressive.

The management of acute radiation effects

At the dose levels necessary to treat carcinoma of the cervix with curative intent, the intestinal mucosa, the cells of which are replaced every three to six days, is usually affected. Most patients develop diarrhoea, which becomes apparent in the second or third week of treatment. With fraction sizes of 1.8–2 Gy, diarrhoea can usually be controlled by a low roughage diet and codeine phosphate, without any disruption of treatment. In severe cases, when diarrhoea cannot be controlled or if there is the passage of copious mucus or blood, fraction size may have to be reduced or treatment suspended. Very occasionally, patients will need admission for fluid and electrolyte replacement.

Radiation cystitis occurs less commonly than bowel disturbance and must be distinguished from infection. Treatment of any infection, the maintenance of a high urine output and of an alkaline pH, with administration of oral potassium citrate, may help to relieve symptoms.

Skin reactions are unusual with megavoltage radiotherapy, except when the vulva, with its very thin epidermis, is included in the field. This is because the maximum deposition of energy is below the skin surface and the use of multiple treatment fields reduces the dose to any particular area of skin. Epidermal cells reproduce every two to three weeks and so damage only becomes apparent after that time. Erythema may be followed by dry desquamation or, with more severe damage, by moist desquamation. The basal cells are usually spared, allowing the skin to regrow. Topical steroids may help before the skin is broken, but once this has happened soothing lotions and antibacterials may be necessary.

The bone marrow is very sensitive to radiation and frequent blood counts are essential when large volumes of marrow are included in the treatment fields, as for example when the para-aortic nodes are treated with radiotherapy. The white blood count and the platelet count are affected early whereas anaemia occurs later because of the longer life span of red blood cells.

In premenopausal women, even small doses of radiation to the pelvis will cause sterility and ovarian failure but HRT can be given to most of these women without affecting prognosis.

The management of late radiation effects

Severe late radiation effects should not occur in more than 2–5% of patients treated with radical radiotherapy.

The bowel

The bowel is the most commonly affected organ. This is usually due to external radiotherapy but intracavitary therapy can cause local radiation problems because of the high dose delivered close to normal structures, such as the bladder and rectum. The correct positioning of applicators and reduction of dose in high dose rate insertions should make severe complications rare.

The bowel habit may be permanently altered as a result of increased bowel motility and decreased water absorption. This results in loose and more frequent stools. Some patients are unable to tolerate roughage or fats and require help with their diet. Other measures that can help are regular codeine phosphate or other drugs that decrease intestinal motility. Occasionally, Questran, which binds to bile acids in the bowel, is helpful. More rarely treatment for malabsorption of vitamin B_{12} or folate from the terminal ileum may be needed if there is an increasing mean corpuscular volume (MCV), anaemia or, very occasionally, neurological signs. Rectal bleeding may result from either ulceration or telangiectasia. Treatment of rectal bleeding is with steroid enemas and, occasionally, tranexamic acid. If these measures do not work a defunctioning colostomy may be required. Stenosis leading to obstruction usually affects the small bowel and can be present at more than one level. Surgery to remove the affected bowel is skilled as the vascularity of the irradiated bowel is often very poor, making the healing of anastomoses difficult.

The bladder

Late damage to the bladder may result in a small capacity bladder. This can be caused by late fibrosis or by neurological disturbance resulting in lower pressures within the bladder triggering the desire to micturate. Haematuria, from the telangiectasia in the bladder lining, may be mild or sufficiently severe to need urinary diversion. Haematuria can be triggered by infection and treatment of the infection is often sufficient to stop the bleeding. Patients with this problem should be encouraged to increase their fluid intake. A high urinary output can help prevent repeated infections by keeping the bladder 'washed out'. Tranexamic acid may reduce the frequency and severity of bleeding and the occurrence of 'clot retention'.

Before making a diagnosis of radiation damage in patients complaining of bleeding from either the rectum or bladder, full investigations need to be carried out to rule out recurrent tumour.

The vagina

The most common problem affecting the vagina from both external and intracavitary radiation is dryness and shortening but HRT or local oestrogen creams can help prevent this. Rarely superficial necrosis of the vaginal mucosa can occur and if radiation damage is severe, necrosis of the bladder base or rectal wall can result in fistula formation.

Other late radiation effects

Other rare late manifestations of radiation damage include *ureteric stenosis*, although this is usually due to recurrent tumour, *avascular necrosis of the femoral heads*, more commonly seen in the days before megavoltage radiotherapy, and *lower limb oedema*. The latter is seldom due to radiotherapy alone and is often a symptom of recurrent tumour in the pelvis or deep-vein thrombosis. It does, however, occur more frequently when the patient has received a combination of surgery and radiotherapy.

References

Brenner, D. J. and Hall, E. J. (1991). Fractionated high dose versus low dose rate regimens for intracavitary brachytherapy of the cervix. 1: General considerations based on radiobiology. *British Journal of Radiology*, **64**, 133–41.

Fu, K. K. and Phillips, T. L. (1990). High dose-rate versus low dose-rate intracavitary brachytherapy for carcinoma of the cervix. *International Journal of Radiation, Oncology, Biology, Physics*, **19**, 791–6.

Harrington, K. J., Lambert, H. E., Price, G. D. *et al.*. (1994). The use of cervagem to induce dilation prior to intracavitary radiotherapy for carcinoma of the cervix. *International Journal of Gynecological Cancer*, **4**, 404–7.

Hunter, R. D. (1995). The Manchester experience with LDR variation in brachytherapy of cervix carcinoma. In *International brachytherapy, Abstracts of the 8th International Brachytherapy Conference*, pp. 52–5. Nice, France.

Khoury, G. G., Bulman, A. S., and Joslin, C. A. F. (1991). Long term results of Cathetron high dose rate intracavitary radiotherapy in the treatment of carcinoma of the cervix. *British Journal of Radiology*, **64**, 1036–43.

Orner, J., Shin, K., and Ho, A. (1996). Principles of radiation therapy. In *Handbook of gynecological oncology* (2nd edn), (ed. M. S. Piver), pp. 248–74. Little, Brown and Co, Boston.

Sharma, S. C., Patel, F. D., Gupta, B. D. *et al.* (1991). Clinical trial of LDR versus HDR brachytherapy in carcinoma of the cervix. Report of the 6th International Selectron Users Meeting. *Selectron Brachytherapy Journal*, 5, 75–9.

Trott, N. G. (1987). Radionuclides in brachytherapy: radium and after. *British Journal of Radiology, Suppl.* 21.

Further reading

Dische, S. (1995). Clinical radiobiology. In *Treatment of cancer* (3rd edn) (ed. P. Price and K. Sikora), pp. 57–72. Chapman and Hall, London.

10

Chemotherapy

Introduction

The use of chemotherapy in gynaecological cancer is increasing. It can be given with either curative or palliative intent, or as an adjunct to surgery or radiotherapy. Chemotherapy is the definitive treatment for the rare germ cell and trophoblastic tumours where it gives rise to high cure rates. However, its major role is non-curative, as in the management of advanced and recurrent gynaecological cancers, especially of the ovary.

Adjuvant chemotherapy, that is chemotherapy given following either definitive surgery or radiotherapy, is used in particular for post-operative treatment of most epithelial ovarian cancers and has resulted in a prolongation of median survival, but has not increased the five-year survival rate.

Neo-adjuvant chemotherapy is given prior to surgery or radiotherapy to reduce tumour bulk. It has shown some promise in advanced ovarian cancer and equivocal results in studies in advanced cervical cancer. It has also been used for vulvar cancer.

Concomitant chemotherapy and radiotherapy is being increasingly used for advanced cervical and vulvar carcinomas but the benefit of chemotherapy in this setting, in comparison to radiotherapy alone, has not yet been clearly identified and the technique should be regarded as experimental and the subject of carefully controlled trials. In addition, there is a danger of increased toxicity to normal tissues when radiotherapy and chemotherapy are given at the same time and, with radiosensitizing drugs such as 5-fluorouracil or cisplatin, the doses of the combined modalities have to be carefully considered.

Action of cytotoxic drugs

Cytotoxic drugs damage all dividing cells, both normal and malignant. They can be used to treat cancer because normal cells are better at repairing the damage caused by the drugs. Some cells that divide rapidly, such as those of the bone marrow and the bowel mucosa, are particularly susceptible to chemotherapy, so that intervals between treatment courses are necessary to allow repair and regeneration of these normal tissues. Although some cancer cells will also recover between treatments, with the correct dose and timing of treatment, there will be a greater loss of malignant cells than normal cells where treatment is effective. The proliferation of tumour cells is to some extent under the control of autocrine factors produced by the tumour cells themselves and of paracrine factors produced by the surrounding stroma. Tumours do not proliferate at a constant rate. Initially, there appears to be an exponential growth rate with a large growth fraction (the proportion of cells within a population that is actively proliferating) but as the tumour enlarges the growth rate falls, as does the growth fraction, giving a longer doubling time. This appears to be due to cell differentiation or cell death through loss of blood supply or nutrients (Steward *et al.* 1995). In tumours which are clinically detectable (i.e. 1 cm in each dimension), the growth pattern is as shown in the Gompertzian growth curve (Fig. 10.1).

The shorter the doubling time of a tumour when treatment is started the better the response to chemotherapy. This is because the response to chemotherapy is dependent on the number of cells synthesizing DNA in a growing stage. Larger tumours with a low proliferation rate will respond less well to chemotherapy but as the tumour gets smaller with treatment, the proliferation rate will increase.

The cell cycle

All cells during their lifetime go through a cell cycle. Chemotherapeutic agents act at various phases of this cycle. This action can be specific to one phase, that is *cell cycle stage specific (phase specific)*, or occur at any time during the cycle, that is *cell cycle stage non-specific (cycle specific)*.

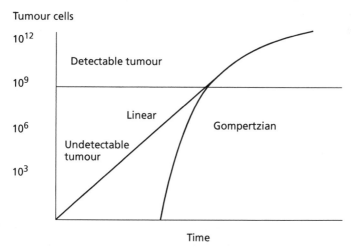

Fig. 10.1 The Gompertzian curve in gynaecological cancer.

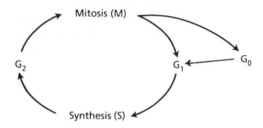

Fig. 10.2 Phases of the cell cycle.

The phases of the cell cycle are mitosis (M) when cell division takes place, leading to G_1, an intermitotic phase when the cell is preparing for cell DNA synthesis. DNA synthesis takes place in the S phase when DNA is copied in preparation for cell division. The G_2 phase follows the S phase when the cell prepares for mitosis. In mitosis the cell divides into two daughter cells. Following mitosis cells either go back into the cell cycle to go through all the phases again or go into a resting phase, G_0 (Fig. 10.2). Cells in G_0 are resistant to chemotherapeutic drugs which are cell cycle stage specific, but they are not resistant to those which are cell cycle stage non-specific.

Hypotheses to explain cytotoxic action

Several hypotheses have been formulated to explain the action of cytotoxic therapy and cell kill. Skipper *et al.* (1964) working with the L1210 leukaemia in mice concluded that: (1) the survival of an animal is inversely related to its tumour burden; (2) a single leukaemic cell can multiply sufficiently to kill the host; (3) a given dose of a drug kills a constant *fraction* not a constant number of cells; (4) for most drugs there is a relationship between the dose of the drug and the elimination of tumour cells. This means that tumours are best treated when they are small and must continue to be treated even when they are no longer detectable in order to kill all the cancer cells.

Norton and Simon (1977) considered that to overcome the slower rate of regression of a tumour as it decreases in size with chemotherapy but, according to the rules of the Gompertzian growth curve (Fig. 10.1), has an increasing growth rate, an increase in intensity of treatment is necessary. This can be by increasing the dosage of drugs after initial treatment or by switching to new drugs.

Goldie and Coldman (1979) produced a mathematical model to explain the development of resistance to cytotoxic chemotherapy. This suggested that populations of cells could randomly become resistant to chemotherapeutic agents. The theoretical extension of their hypothesis supports the use of multiple non-cross resistant drugs given simultaneously in combination regimens.

While these hypotheses are of interest and can form a basis for designing chemotherapy regimens there is no evidence that they apply to all cases of cancer.

Testing new drugs

Many compounds are tested *in vitro*, using human cell lines, to find active agents for treating cancer. Those shown to have activity *in vitro* undergo clinical testing in three phases (Table 10.1): (1) to establish the maximum tolerated dose (MTD) in humans; (2) the range of antitumour activity of the new drug; and (3) to compare the new drug either alone or in combination, with the standard treatment for a particular tumour. Drug toxicity is evaluated in all these phases. If these studies are successful the drug will be licensed for availability on prescription but post-marketing surveillance continues.

Considerable effort is expended on searching for new cytotoxic drugs, which involves lengthy development time and high cost to ensure their safety.

Pharmacology

When considering the use of a cytotoxic drug the methods of absorption, distribution, metabolism, excretion, and penetration into the tumour, must all be taken into account. Penetration of the drug will depend on the size, vascularization, and site of the tumour. In most situations it is considered that 'drug exposure', as measured by the area under the concentration–time curve (AUC) at the tumour site, is the crucial determinant of drug activity (Steward *et al.* 1995).

Table 10.1 Phases of development of a cytotoxic therapy

Phase I	Patients with a range of relapsed/recurrent tumours are treated with escalating doses of the test drug to determine the maximum tolerated dose (MTD) in humans. The profile of drug toxicity is noted. Assessable disease is not required, although disease response is noted where possible
Phase II	Patients with certain tumour types (usually those that have been shown to be responsive in phase I studies) receive a number of courses of test drug to define the spectrum of its antitumour activity. Further assessment of drug toxicity is performed. These patients usually have relapsed disease and have already received a number of different therapies
Phase III	Patients with certain tumour type(s) are randomly allocated to receive either standard therapy (control) or the test agent. Detailed assessment of toxicity is conducted
'Phase IV'	Post-marketing surveillance of the drug

Only a few drugs have predictable bioavailability from absorption from the intestinal tract to enable them to be given orally, therefore the majority of cytotoxic drugs are given by the parenteral, usually intravenous, route.

The metabolism of many of the cytotoxic drugs within the body has not been fully described. Some are metabolized in the liver and are excreted in the bile. Cyclophosphamide is not active until it reaches the liver as it requires activation by hepatic enzymes which convert it into its cytotoxic form. Other cytotoxic drugs, such as the anthracyclines and the vinca alkaloids are excreted as active agents, via the liver, in the bile. All such drugs will need to be used at a reduced dose in the presence of impaired hepatic function. Most cytotoxic drugs are excreted in the urine. Impaired renal function will delay this excretion resulting in increased toxicity and this is of particular importance in drugs, such as cisplatin, which are nephrotoxic.

It is important that before deciding on dosage for each patient, both liver and renal function are assessed as well as marrow function. Marrow function is affected by cytotoxic therapy in view of the fast turnover of its cells and needs to be within acceptable limits before each treatment course, if severe morbidity is to be avoided. Those patients at risk of increased toxicity from poor renal or hepatic function, will have their drug dosage modified according to their ability to metabolize and eliminate the drug.

Few drugs cross the blood–brain barrier, although exceptions include carmustine, etoposide, methotrexate, and ifosfamide. This barrier can be overcome by intrathecal administration, usually with methotrexate, but the need for this in the treatment of gynaecological cancer is rare.

Interactions of cytotoxic drugs

The majority of patients receiving cytotoxic chemotherapy will also receive a range of other drugs during the course of their treatment. Interactions between cytotoxic and non-cytotoxic drugs may occur. Cisplatin must not be administered at the same time as aminoglycoside antibiotics, as both can cause nephrotoxicity and ototoxicity, or with thiazide diuretics as renal tubular damage may result. Warfarin concentrations may be altered by the simultaneous administration of methotrexate or medroxyprogesterone acetate, leading to difficulty in anticoagulant control. Steroids can increase the need for diabetic control. Specialist advice from the pharmacist should always be obtained if a patient is on multiple medication when chemotherapy is planned.

Classification of cytotoxic drugs

Cytotoxic drugs can be divided into separate groups each with a similar mode of action at the cellular level (Fig. 10.3). These are the *alkylating agents*, the *antitumour antibiotics*, the *antimetabolites*, the *vinca alkaloids*, the *podophyllotoxins*, the *taxanes*, and *miscellaneous agents*.

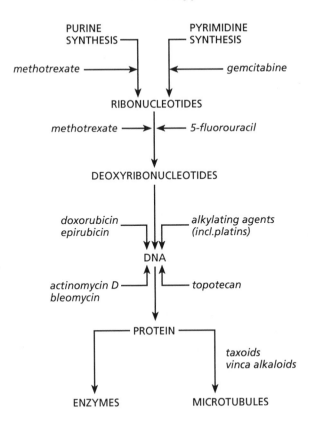

Fig. 10.3 Sites of action at cellular level of commonly used cytotoxic agents in gynaecological cancer.

Cytotoxic drugs used in treating gynaecological cancer

Alkylating agents

Alkylating agents are so called because they have alkyl groups that bond to amino or carboxyl groups on nucleic acids. The main mechanism of cytotoxicity results from this binding to bases in the DNA, preventing cell replication. The most commonly used alkylating agents for gynaecological cancers are the platinum drugs, cyclophosphamide, ifosfamide and to a lesser extent, treosulfan, and the oral alkylating agents, chlorambucil and melphalan.

Platinum agents

Cisplatin This agent, alone or in combination, is used in the treatment of most gynaecological tumours. The overall response rate in epithelial tumours is approximately 70 percent, and germ cell tumours are also highly sensitive. Cisplatin is the most active single agent for cervical cancer with a response rate in recurrent disease of about 40 percent. It is also active in endometrial carcinoma.

Cisplatin is given intravenously at a dose of 70–100 mg/m^2 when given as a single agent, and 50 mg/m^2 in combination. Cisplatin has an initial half-life of 40 minutes and a second clearance phase of 60 hours. Excretion is via the kidneys.

The most serious side-effect is nephrotoxicity which can worsen during a course of treatment. Precautions which are necessary to reduce this damage to a minimum are discussed later in this chapter under 'renal tract toxicity' (p. 226). Neurotoxicity, mainly peripheral neuropathy, appears to be dose-related. The symptoms of tingling or numbness in the fingers or toes can persist for many months after the cessation of treatment and with very high doses may be irreversible (p. 228). Ototoxicity, with some loss of high tone hearing, occurs quite commonly. Nausea and vomiting is a serious problem with cisplatin as it can be severe and last for several days. For the treatment of these gastrointestinal symptoms see under 'nausea and vomiting' (p. 226, and Table 10.2). Myelotoxocity and alopecia are not usually features of treatment with cisplatin.

Carboplatin   This is an analogue of cisplatin and acts in the same manner. At standard dosage it has the advantage of causing minimal nephrotoxicity and neurotoxocity. Nausea and vomiting are usually easier to control than with cisplatin. However, unlike cisplatin, carboplatin is myelotoxic and low platelet counts are a particular problem as they can occur early in a course of treatment and be sufficiently severe to require support with platelet

Table 10.2 Regimens for nausea and vomiting

Severity	Suggested regimen
Mild/moderate (e.g. carboplatin)	Dexamethasone 8 mg iv bolus stat; *plus* iv 5HT$_3$ antagonist (e.g. 8 mg Ondansetron) for subsequent courses *if emesis occurs*; *plus* metoclopramide 20 mg or domperidone 20 mg orally 3 times daily for 2 days
Severe (e.g. cisplatin)	Dexamethasone 8 mg iv bolus stat 5HT$_3$ antagonist iv stat Repeat at 8–12 hours if necessary; *plus* metoclopromide 20 mg 3 times daily and dexamethasone 2 mg 3 times daily for 2–5 days

infusions. Myelotoxicity appears to be related to renal function and in the presence of impaired renal function, as measured by EDTA or creatinine clearance, a dose reduction is necessary. Carboplatin is excreted in the urine at a constant rate and, therefore, the dose can be calculated from Calvert's formula (Calvert *et al.* 1987), based on the linear relationship between plasma clearance and glomerular filtration rate (GFR). This uses the area under the curve (AUC) of free carboplatin plasma dose concentration versus time. An AUC factor of 5–9 given every 3 weeks is the usual dose. This formula allows patients with normal renal indices to receive high doses of carboplatin more safely than when prescribed by surface area.

For a *minimum* dose of carboplatin (AUC 5) the dose is calculated as:

5 (measured clearance [e.g. EDTA] + 25) mg.

Previously, if clearance could not be measured by an excretion test, it could be estimated using the Cockroft-Gault formula (Cockroft and Gault, 1976), which predicts creatinine clearance from serum creatinine, age and weight. However, algorithmic methods of estimating creatinine clearance, such as this, may not be reliable at the extremes of age and weight and may not reflect actual clearance, particularly if this is changing rapidly. In addition, these formulae may not take into account the different ratios of muscle mass to total body weight in males and females and may over-estimate clearance in women. For these reasons the use of the Cockroft-Gault formula is not recommended other than to establish that a measured clearance rate is not changing with consequtive courses of chemotherapy.

Table 10.3 gives doses of carboplatin based on GFR to achieve an AUC of 5 or 6. Carboplatin is as effective as cisplatin in the treatment of ovarian and endometrial cancers but appears to be less effective than cisplatin for

Table 10.3 Carboplatin dose based on glomerular filtration rate (GFR)

GFR (ml/min)	Carboplatin dose (mg) Dose based on measured clearance
50	375
60	425
70	475
80	525
90	575
100	625
110	675

Measured clearance using EDTA clearance and renogram: 5 (EDTA clearance +25) mg cervical cancer. As there is minimal nephrotoxicity a forced diuresis is not required and carboplatin can therefore be given, as an outpatient, in a 60-minute infusion.

Other platinum agents   Other analogues of cisplatin are under investigation including one that can be administered orally.

Cyclophosphamide and ifosfamide

Cyclophosphamide, an oxazophosphorene alkylating agent, was one of the earliest cytotoxic drugs used in cancer therapy and is still in use. Ifosfamide is an analogue of cyclophosphamide which is less myelosuppressive. Both are active drugs in gynaecological cancer. Cyclophosphamide is well absorbed by mouth but is more usually given in high dose intravenously. Both drugs are activated in the liver by the cytochrome P450 system, producing active metabolites which are excreted in the urine where they can cause a chemical cystitis. The latter can be largely prevented by the co-administration of uromitexan (Mesna) (see p. 227). The oral dose of cyclophosphamide is usually 100 mg/m^2 daily. Peak concentration is reached in 1 hour and the half-life is 5–6 hours. Intravenously, the dose can vary from 750 mg/m^2 to 1.5 gm/m^2 or even higher when bone marrow support, with a transplant or stem cell infusion, is required. Ifosfamide is usually given at a dose of 5 gm/m^2 over 24 hours with Mesna.

Apart from being toxic to the urothelium, both drugs cause alopecia and are myelotoxic. Ifosfamide can cause encephalopathy resulting in somnolence, confusion, and coma.

Treosulfan

Treosulfan is a bifunctional alkylating agent which has been found to be effective in ovarian cancer. It is used both as adjuvant therapy following surgery and in palliative and refractory disease as little, if any, cross-resistance has been reported between treosulfan and other cytotoxic drugs. Treosulfan is well absorbed by mouth so it can be given orally in intermittent courses, although it is usually given intravenously in an infusion over 10 minutes. It is excreted via the kidneys. The recommended dose of treosulfan, by the intravenous route, is 7 gm/m^2, every 4 weeks. The main adverse reaction of treosulfan is marrow depression. Gastrointestinal problems, such as nausea, vomiting, and abdominal pain, can occur when treosulfan is given orally but are rare when the drug is given intravenously.

Chlorambucil and melphalan

For many years an oral alkylating agent, such as chlorambucil or melphalan, was the main treatment available for patients with inoperable cancer of the ovary. Few lasting responses were seen. Their role is now minimal and they are usually given as primary treatment in elderly patients considered unfit for any other chemotherapy or as second-line treatment, although their record in this latter situation is poor. Both drugs are toxic to the bone marrow having a cumulative effect and therefore need to be given in intermittent courses to allow the bone marrow to recover. A usual dose of chlorambucil is 10 mg daily for 10–14 days per month, and 10 mg daily for 7 days every 6 weeks for melphalan. Treatment longer than one year can give rise to acute myeloid leukaemia.

Hexamethylmelamine

Hexamethylmelamine is an aziridine alkylating agent. It is absorbed well from the bowel and therefore is given orally, usually as second-line therapy for ovarian cancer as it has some activity even when the platinum drugs have failed, suggesting that it is non cross-resistant. It tends to cause nausea and vomiting, diarrhoea, and leucopenia. Rarely, central nervous toxicity can occur.

Cytotoxic antibiotics

Many of these drugs behave in a similar fashion to alkylating agents causing cross-linkage between DNA and RNA strands in the cell. They also act as intercalating agents, free radical generators, and chelators of trace metals.

Anthracyclines

Doxorubicin (Adriamycin), an anthracycline which is used in gynaecological cancer, comes from the *Streptomyces* fungus. Doxorubicin can affect cardiac muscle. The semi-synthetic analogue, epirubicin, which is considered to be less cardiotoxic appears to be equally effective. Doxorubicin is not cycle stage-specific but it acts mainly in the S phase of the cell cycle by binding to nucleic acids, thus inhibiting DNA and RNA synthesis. Doxorubicin is used for ovarian epithelial tumours in combination chemotherapy regimens, for example, CAP (cyclophosphamide, doxorubicin, cisplatin). It also has a therapeutic role in the management of endometrial carcinomas and uterine sarcomas. Doxorubicin is given by the intravenous route in a fast-running drip as great care has to be taken that it does not extravasate causing a severe and painful reaction which often proceeds to a chronic skin ulcer requiring plastic surgery. The anthracyclines are metabolized in the liver and excreted in the bile and so are contra-indicated in the presence of severe liver damage. The dose of doxorubicin is usually 50–75 mg/m^2 every 3 weeks, when given as a single agent.

Doxorubicin is a very toxic drug which affects the bone marrow and causes total alopecia of head hair unless scalp cooling is used. It also produces mucositis and severe nausea and vomiting, the latter being ameliorated by the use of 5HT$_3$ antagonists. Its cardiotoxicity, mentioned earlier, limits the safe *total* dose of doxorubicin to 450 mg/m^2 as higher doses increase the possibility of cardiomyopathy, which is frequently fatal (see p. 230). For epirubicin the dose is 75–100 mg/m^2, every 3 weeks to a maximum cumulative dose of 0.9–1 g/m^2, to avoid cardiotoxicity.

Bleomycin

Bleomycin is a synthetic antibiotic originally isolated from *Streptomyces verticillus* but is now chemically synthesized. It acts mainly in the premitotic (G$_2$) phase. It is usually given by intravenous infusion but can also be given subcutaneously, by intramuscular injection or into the pleural cavity, the latter to treat malignant effusions. It is mainly used in gynaecological cancer in the treatment of germ cell tumours but it is also incorporated in some combination regimens for treating cervical cancer.

Bleomycin causes little marrow suppression, unlike the majority of cytotoxic agents. Dermatological effects include pigmentation and thickening of the skin especially in skin creases and areas of trauma. Hypersensitivity reactions can occur but can be largely prevented by giving the drug as a 24-hour intravenous infusion at a dose of 15–30 units daily rather than as a bolus and also by the simultaneous administration of steroids. The most serious toxicity of bleomycin is that it can cause progressive pulmonary fibrosis particularly in the elderly. This is dose-related and therefore the dose of bleomycin is dependent on age. If the patient is over 80 years of age the dose is 15 units weekly, to a maximum of 100 units, increasing to 30 units weekly for those aged 70–79 years to a total of 200 units, and in younger patients the dose is 200–300 units given at a rate of 30–60 units weekly. The cumulative dose is rarely allowed to exceed 300 units. Lung function must be measured before starting treatment with bleomycin and regularly through the course of therapy. Reductions in transfer factor of carbon monoxide are an indication to stop treatment. Basal crepitations or an abnormal chest X-ray are also indications to stop bleomycin.

Mitomycin C

This drug, isolated from the *Streptomyces caespitosus*, which acts by both cross-linking and alkylating DNA, is used in gynaecological cancer as part of a combination regimen for the treatment of cancer of the cervix and vulva. The main toxicity is to the bone marrow, particularly to the platelet precursors. Bone marrow suppression is delayed so treatment is only given every 6 weeks and the dose is usually 10 mg/m^2.

Actinomycin D

Actinomycin D is another drug isolated from the *Streptomyces* species, and is useful in treating rare tumours such as sarcomas, germ cell tumours, and choriocarcinomas. Actinomycin D is cell cycle specific, acting mainly in G$_1$

and S phases. It is myelotoxic and increases the sensitivity of tissues to radiation. The drug is usually used in combination chemotherapy and is given intravenously at a dose of 15 μg/kg.

Antimetabolites

Antimetabolites are analogues of nucleic acid bases that compete with the normal metabolites that are necessary for enzymes involved in DNA and RNA synthesis.

Methotrexate

Methotrexate is a folic acid antagonist and interferes with the formation of DNA and RNA in the nucleus. It acts by inhibiting the enzyme, dihydro-folate reductase, which is a catalyst for the conversion of folic acid to its active tetrahydrofolate metabolites, which are necessary for the synthesis of DNA and RNA. Methotrexate is mainly active in the S phase of the cell cycle. It is active against squamous carcinomas and in trophoblastic disease.

Methotrexate can be given orally but with doses greater than 100 mg it is usually given intravenously. After intravenous injection there is an initial half-life of 45 minutes, a 3-hour period of renal excretion, and then a very long terminal half-life, accounting for its toxicity. The main toxic effects are on the bone marrow, bowel, and mucous membranes. Pneumonitis is occasionally induced. These effects are reversed by rescue with folinic acid, which bypasses the enzyme block caused by the methotrexate. The folinic acid rescue, given orally or intravenously, is commenced 24 hours after the start of methotrexate administration, for all doses over 50 mg. Without this rescue, high dose methotrexate, with its prolonged half-life, would cause fatal toxicity. Inadequate rescue, with folinic acid being given for too short a period, results in oral mucositis and occasionally conjunctivitis. This is avoided by continuing folinic acid administration until the serum concentration of methotrexate, measured daily, is below 10^{-7} M. Methotrexate should be avoided in the presence of marked ascites or large pleural effusions as it tends to accumulate at these sites which will delay its excretion, leading to myelosuppression.

Methotrexate is excreted in the urine and with large doses, unless preventive measures are taken (p. 227), crystals can be deposited in the renal tubules causing renal failure. Methotrexate should not be given in the presence of renal failure. Rarely, methotrexate given as a bolus, can also cause liver damage.

Methotrexate is strongly bound to albumin and can be displaced by other protein-binding agents, for example, phenytoin, anticoagulants, salicylates, sulfonamides, tetracycline, and acidic anti-inflammatory agents, resulting in higher levels of free methotrexate and increased toxicity.

5-Fluorouracil (5FU)

5-Flourouracil is a pyrimidine analogue that competes with uracil deoxy-riboside on the enzyme thymidilate synthetase necessary for DNA synthesis. 5FU is not cell cycle stage specific but its maximum effect is in the S phase of the cell cycle. This antimetabolite can be given orally but is more reliably administered intravenously. However, as its half-life is only 15 minutes, it is most active when given as a continuous intravenous infusion, using a pump, or when it is combined with folinic acid which prolongs its action. 5FU has some activity in ovarian cancer where it is usually given in combination, and as a radiosensitizer either alone or in combination with cisplatin or mito-mycin C, in cervical and vulval cancer. The main toxicity of 5FU is to the bowel mucosa causing mucositis and diarrhoea when given in large, pro-longed doses. A 'hand-foot' syndrome, known as palmar plantar syndrome, in which the patient complains of painful reddened extremities, can occur with continuous infusion.

Gemcitabine

Gemcitabine (2',2'-difluorodeoxycytidine), a pyrimidine antimetabolite, is a new drug that has been shown to be active in gynaecological cancer. Responses have been obtained in ovarian cancer resistant to platinum drugs and it also appears to be promising as a radiosensitizer for the treatment of cervical cancer. The main toxicities are marrow depression, nausea and vomiting, and diarrhoea.

Vinca alkaloids

Vincristine and vinblastine are extracts from the periwinkle plant, *Catharanthus roseus*. These drugs act during mitosis by binding to tubulin, a spindle protein. The toxicity of vincristine is mainly neurological. It can cause a troublesome peripheral sensory neuropathy and occasionally paralytic ileus but it has almost no effect on bone marrow. Extravasation can result in tissue damage. In contrast to vincristine the toxicity of vin-blastine is mainly to the bone marrow. Both drugs cause some alopecia. The vinca alkaloids are mainly used in gynaecological cancer as part of a combination regimen for germ cell tumours.

Podophyllotoxins

These are semi-synthetic drugs derived from *Podophyllin peltatum*. Etoposide, a topoisomerase II inhibitor, also known as VP16 and epipodophyllotoxin, is cell cycle stage specific preventing cells from entering mitosis. It is well-absorbed orally although somewhat unpredictably. It is used in combination in the treatment of both germ cell tumours and gestational trophoblastic disease and, as a single agent, has some activity in relapsed ovarian cancer.

The taxanes

This class of compounds, also known as taxoids, acts by a novel mechanism which results in the stabilization of microtubules that are essential cellular components needed for various cellular activities including mitosis. Paclitaxel comes from the bark of the Pacific yew tree, *Taxus brevifolia*, and docetaxel is a semi-synthetic taxane developed from the needles of the European yew tree, *Taxus baccate*. The taxanes enhance microtubule assembly and inhibit depolymerization of tubulin. This leads to the formation of bundles of microtubules in the cell which blocks the formation and division of the normal mitotic spindle with arrest in G^2 and M phases of the cell cycle. This action prevents the cell from dividing. The two most commonly used taxanes are paclitaxel and docetaxel. Both drugs bind to serum proteins and there is minimal urinary excretion. Body clearance is dependent on metabolism, biliary excretion and/or distribution, and tissue binding (Gelmon 1994). Both paclitaxel and docetaxel have considerable activity in ovarian cancer with paclitaxel, at present, being the most frequently used. The clinical role of paclitaxel and docetaxel is discussed in Chapter 2 on ovarian cancer.

In addition to myelosuppression and sensory neuropathy, which can occur even after the first dose of treatment, paclitaxel can cause severe hypersensitivity. Patients must be pretreated with a combination of corticosteroids and H_1 and H_2 receptor antagonists (Table 10.4), and close observation is required during the first hour of treatment. Severe reactions include dyspnoea, severe hypotension, angio-oedema, and generalized urticaria. This occurs in approximately 2 percent of patients despite premedication. Myelosuppression, mainly neutropenia, is common and dose-limiting but anaemia, although also occurring frequently, is seldom severe. Thrombocytopenia can also be present. Peripheral neuropathy causes paraesthesia in the majority of patients but is seldom severe enough at standard dosage, to warrant a reduction in dose. It usually resolves within a few months of stopping treatment.

Rarely, cardiac conduction abnormalities occur including arrhythmias and cardiac conduction defects but these are almost always asymptomatic.

Table 10.4 Premedication for paclitaxel chemotherapy

Time prior to paclitaxel	Drug and dose
12 hours	Dexamethasone 20 mg orally
6 hours	Dexamethasone 20 mg orally
30 minutes	Chlorpheniramine (H_1 receptor antagonist) 10 mg iv in 5–10 ml normal saline
	Ranitidine 50 mg iv; *or* cimetidine (H_2 receptor antagonist) 300 mg in 20 ml of normal saline given over 2 minutes

Probably the most distressing side-effect for the patient is alopecia which is not only total but also affects hair all over the body, not only that of the head.

Docitaxel has a similar toxicity pattern to paclitaxel but in addition it can cause skin reactions and oedema.

In Europe, paclitaxel is given at a dose of 175 mg/m^2, over 3 hours, in 500 ml of 5 percent dextrose at 3-weekly intervals following premedication to prevent hypersensitivity (Table 10.4). In America the standard dose is 135 mg/m^2 over 24 hours. A suggestion under investigation is that paclitaxel is most active when the treatment infusion is prolonged (96 hours). Bone marrow depression is less with the 3-hour infusion compared to the 24-hour infusion, and early reports failed to show any reduction in efficacy for the shorter infusion period (ten Bookkel Huinink *et al.* 1993).

Miscellaneous drugs

Topoisomerase inhibitor: Topotecan

Topotecan is a topoisomerase I inhibitor (a nuclear enzyme essential for DNA synthesis), which is under investigation. It has shown activity in both refractory and advanced ovarian cancer for which, as a single agent, it appears to be as effective as paclitaxel. It is given as an intravenous infusion and its main toxicity is to the bone marrow.

Metalloproteinase inhibitors

These new drugs, of which the orally active Marimastat is an example, are being investigated in advanced and recurrent ovarian cancer. They act by inhibiting matrix metalloproteinases which are thought to promote the growth and dissemination of tumours.

Route of administration

Oral

Only a few drugs, mainly alkylating agents, such as chlorambucil and etoposide, are well absorbed from the gastrointestinal tract. Administration is usually in pulsed courses of 7–14 days in each month. The interval between courses allows normal tissues, in particular the bone marrow, to recover.

Systemic

Most cytotoxic drugs are given intravenously at intervals of one to four weeks. Some drugs are given as bolus injections to achieve a high peak for a short period of time, whereas others (e.g. 5-fluorouracil) are more effective if infused over several hours or days to give a low but prolonged concentration in the body. In these instances the drug is given through a central line using portable syringe pumps, thus allowing improved quality of life for the patient.

Many cytotoxic drugs are intensely irritant and must be administered intravenously either well diluted or as a bolus in a fast-running drip. The drugs should always be washed through with normal saline after administration to avoid sclerosis of the veins, which will make successive courses harder to give. It is important to avoid extravasation by ensuring that the cannula or needle is located within the vein, by observing some back-flow of blood, before giving the drug. Administration should stop if there is any local pain as this suggests that the drug is leaking into tissues. The management of extravasation of cytotoxic drugs is discussed later.

Although seldom used for cytotoxic therapy, intramuscular injection provides a suitable route of administration for a few drugs (e.g. bleomycin), which must be given with lignocaine to reduce muscle pain. Rarely, drugs are given by direct intra-arterial perfusion. As so few drugs cross the blood–brain barrier drugs, such as methotrexate, which are used for treating cerebral-spinal malignancies (e.g. in the treatment of some cases of gestational trophoblastic disease), are instilled directly into the cerebral-spinal fluid (*intrathecal administration*). This may be associated with local complications such as arachnoiditis, acute myelitis, or even a chronic demyelinating encephelopathy.

Intrapleural and intraperitoneal

Chemotherapy can be given into both the pleural and peritoneal cavities. Bleomycin, at a dose of 60 units, has been used in this way for the treatment of recurrent malignant pleural effusions, by acting as a chemical sclerosant stimulating an inflammatory reaction and the formation of adhesions. Non-cytotoxic agents such as tetracycline or talc, are as effective and less systemically toxic.

Intraperitoneal chemotherapy, where cytotoxic drugs are instilled in a peritoneal dialysate, has been carried out as an investigative procedure in ovarian cancer for some years. This allows a very high and prolonged local concentration of the drug in the peritoneum, which is the commonest site of recurrence of ovarian cancer. Penetration of drugs is limited to 1–2 mm from the peritoneal surface. Cisplatin has been the drug of choice as it is one of the few drugs that does not give rise to severe peritoneal reactions, causing abdominal pain and obstructions from adhesions. Most of this work has been with patients found to have minimal residual disease (<5 mm) at second look surgery following initial chemotherapy. However, as previously mentioned in Chapter 2 (p. 32), a Gynecological Oncology Group (GOG) study has compared, as initial chemotherapy in 546 women with stage II ovarian cancer, with residual tumour masses of less than 2 cm, a combination regimen of intravenous cisplatin (100 mg/m^2) and cyclophosphamide (600 mg/m^2) with the same regimen, but with the cisplatin given intraperitoneally. Increased length of survival and decreased toxicity was found in favour of the intraperitoneal route (Alberts *et al.* 1996). Recently, interest has been shown in using paclitaxel as an intraperitoneal drug as it is well tolerated, does not cause adhesions, and gives rise to very high concentration within the peritoneal cavity compared to the systemic dose.

Drug dose

Calculation of dose

To ensure that patients receive an equivalent amount of a cytotoxic drug, regardless of differences in build and weight, the dose of most cytotoxic drugs is based on the surface area of the patient measured in square metres (Fig. 10.4). It is estimated from the patient's height and weight. With carboplatin, which is excreted in a very predictable way, dependent on the glomerular filtration rate (GFR), a formula incorporating the GFR is used instead of surface area. The methods for doing this have been discussed under Carboplatin and the dosage table is shown in Table 10.3.

If, despite using these parameters, a drug proves to be more myelotoxic than is acceptable, the dose is reduced to prevent the occurrence of severe leucopenia or thrombocytopenia or, if dose reduction is considered ill-advised, G-CSF (granulocyte–colony stimulating factor) support is given with the subsequent courses. Dose modification may also be needed if hepatic or renal impairment is present as this may lead to slower metabolism or delayed excretion of the drug.

High dose chemotherapy

The attractive hypothesis is that, by increasing the total dose of a drug, an improved response rate may be obtained. However, randomized studies to date have failed to confirm this. This may be due to the fact that these studies have involved patients with very advanced disease, in whom achievement of the prescribed dose intensity has not been possible. With the very high doses of drugs needed to overcome inherent drug resistance, toxicity becomes a problem and although bone marrow depression can be counteracted by the use of G-CSF support, bone marrow rescue or peripheral stem cell infusion, severe non-haematological morbidity (e.g. peripheral neurotoxicity and nephrotoxicity with cisplatin), becomes the limiting factor.

Duration and scheduling of chemotherapy

Duration

The optimum duration for a course of chemotherapy is unknown. A palpable tumour will contain 10^9–10^{12} cells but even if it shrinks to a

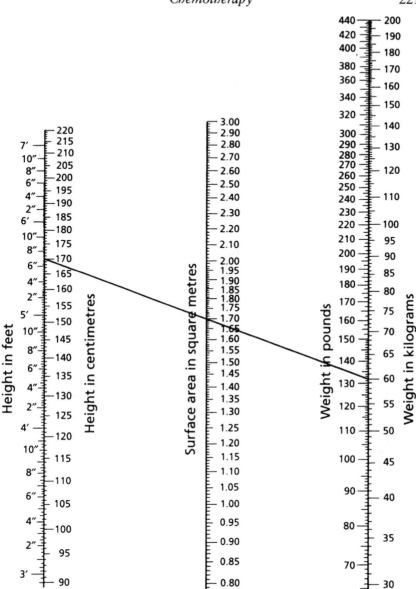

Fig. 10.4 Nomogram for calculating body surface area.

clinically undetectable mass it may contain 10^8 cells and so further chemotherapy is needed (Fig. 10.5). Rarely, when tumours produce a specific tumour marker, such as βhCG in trophoblastic disease and some germ cell tumours, marker measurements allow the treatment period to be

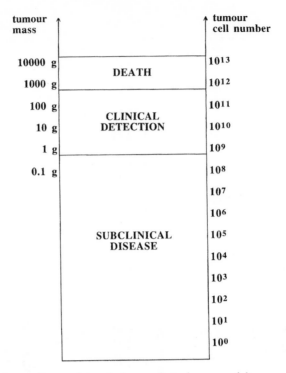

Fig. 10.5 Tumour cell growth in relation to clinical course of disease.

defined accurately for each patient. In the common epithelial tumours, sufficiently sensitive tumour markers to define accurately when to stop treatment do not exist. Even CA125, useful at defining response to chemotherapy in epithelial ovarian tumours, is not sensitive enough to detect small volume disease. Prolonged chemotherapy causes toxicity, especially to the bone marrow, which may become permanently hypoplastic producing a pancytopaenia. The risk of developing a second malignancy, including leukaemia, increases with the higher total doses of cytotoxic drugs. This is especially the case if an alkylating agent is used or if chemotherapy is combined with radiotherapy. In ovarian cancer no benefit has been demonstrated from receiving more than six courses of chemotherapy in the adjuvant setting (Lambert *et al.* 1997).

Scheduling

The importance of scheduling chemotherapy is becoming more apparent. Slevin *et al.* (1989), demonstrated a dramatic differential response to intravenous etoposide for small cell tumour of the lung, when administered as a single or 5-day infusion, with between 10 percent and 90 percent of patients responding, respectively. The increased efficacy of continuous infusion of 5-fluorouracil (5FU) has already been mentioned. The effect of combination chemotherapy with 5FU, cisplatin, and epirubicin given 3-weekly, the 5FU being given as a continuous infusion, has proven to be effective in such tumours as gastric carcinoma previously resistant to similar combination chemotherapy, given as pulsed courses. With many of the older drugs the optimum scheduling for the greatest effect and least toxicity is unknown but this matter is being examined in relation to paclitaxel where 3-hour infusions have been compared to 24-hour infusions, and 24-hour infusions are now being compared to 96-hour infusions.

Combination chemotherapy

The development of resistance by malignant cells to a single cytotoxic agent has encouraged the use of combination chemotherapy regimens with the aim of increasing antitumour activity and reducing or delaying the development of drug resistance. In order to achieve this, the drugs in the combination regimen must all be active against the tumour and have different mechanisms of cellular action and minimally overlapping toxicities (Steward *et al.* 1995 and Fig. 10.3).

Despite the theoretical advantages, combination therapy to date has not proved superior to single agent therapy in the treatment of most gynae-cological malignancies in that, although response rates are increased, survival is unchanged. The exceptions are the rare germ cell tumours and high grade gestational trophoblastic tumours in which multiple drug therapy, given concurrently or sequentially, has led to a high cure rate.

Prevention and management of the toxic effects of chemotherapy

Chemotherapy can cause toxicity ranging from mild to severe. In order to assess the gravity of these side-effects, The Eastern Cooperative Oncology Group (ECOG) has introduced a grading system from 0 to 4 that is now used in most centres. Examples are shown in Table 10.5.

Immune reactions

Some cytotoxic agents, especially bleomycin and paclitaxel, can produce an immune response either by a direct effect on the mast cells in the tissues, which release histamine, or indirectly by production of an IgE antibody. Both of these mechanisms can lead to anaphylactic shock. This is a rare complication and, if it occurs despite preventive measures already detailed under these drugs, it requires immediate treatment with antihistamines: chlorpheniramine, 10–20 mg by slow infection, adrenaline by intramuscular injection or subcutaneously, 0.5–1 mg (0.5–1 ml of 1:1000 solution), every 10 minutes as required, and steroids: dexamethasone.

Table 10.5 ECOG toxicity criteria: haematological and gastrointestinal

	Grade 0	Grade 1	Grade 2	Grade 3	Grade 4
Haematology					
Neutrophils*	> or = 2.0	1.5–1.9	1.0–1.4	0.5–0.9	< 0.5
Leucopenia*	> or = 4.0	3.0–3.9	2.0–2.9	1.0–1.9	< 1.0
Thrombocytopenia*	> or = 100	75–99	50–74	25–40	< 25
Gastrointestinal					
Mucosal/oral	No change	Soreness/erythema	Erythema ulcers: can eat solids	Ulcers: requires liquid diet only	Alimentaton not possible
Nausea/vomiting	None	Nausea	Transient vomiting	Vomiting requiring therapy	Intractable vomiting
Diarrhoea	None	Transient < or = 2 days	Tolerable > 2 days	Intolerable requiring therapy	Haemorrhagic dehydration

* 1000 mm^3

ECOG, Eastern Cooperative Oncology Group.

Normal tissue toxicity

The tissues affected by cytotoxic drugs include:

- bone marrow
- gastrointestinal tract
- kidneys and urothelium
- skin, hair, and mucosa
- reproductive system
- nervous system
- lungs
- heart
- liver
- injection site

A knowledge of the toxic potential of cytotoxic therapy is essential for the safe management of patients. In addition, it is important to realise that patients who are very elderly or who are in poor health will not tolerate full doses of intensive chemotherapy, and only in very exceptional circumstances are cytotoxic drugs given in the presence of infection.

The main toxicities of individual drugs have been described. The management of toxic effects is dependent on both the clinical problem and the causative drug.

Bone marrow suppression

Myelosuppression occurs to some extent with almost all cytotoxic drugs as the rapidly dividing bone marrow stem cells are particularly sensitive. The exceptions are vincristine, bleomycin and, to some extent, cisplatin. The blood count must be checked regularly between and before each course of treatment. In particular, the count is checked when the myelosuppression is at its maximum or *nadir*, usually 10–14 days after treatment. With some drugs, such as mitomycin, the nadir may occur at 4–5 weeks after treatment, therefore the drug is only given 6-weekly.

Severe infections are uncommon if the granulocyte count remains above 0.5×10^9 per litre but patients must be instructed to report if they are unwell or have a pyrexia. If there is evidence of infection together with a low granulocyte count, intravenous antibiotics will be required but blood cultures should be carried out first. Treatment, with broad spectrum antibiotics, needs to be aggressive as infections in these patients can rapidly become life-threatening. Recombinant human colony stimulating factors have a direct effect on the bone marrow stem cells, increasing tolerance to chemotherapy by stimulating the production of neutrophils and by reducing the duration of neutropenia, thus helping to lower the incidence of secondary infections. These stimulating factors include filgrastim, a granulocyte–colony stimulating factor (GCSF) and molgramostim, a granulocyte macrophage–colony stimulating factor (GM-CSF). A further drug, amifostine, reduces the risk of infection related to neutropenia, and may be used to treat patients receiving cisplatin and cyclophosphamide for advanced ovarian cancer.

Infections following cytotoxic chemotherapy can result not only from pathogenic bacteria but also from commensal organisms. Fungal infections may also develop affecting mucosal surfaces or, more seriously, can become systemic.

Platelet counts reach their nadir 1–2 weeks after treatment and usually do not cause problems until they fall below $15 - 20 \times 10^9$ per litre. If spontaneous bleeding occurs, transfusions of fresh platelets are required but the treatment may need to be repeated daily until the bone marrow recovers and the count rises.

Anaemia usually presents only after several courses of chemotherapy have been given because of the long life span of red blood cells. Transfusion may be required if the haemoglobin falls below 10 g/dl. Recently, recombinant human erythropoeitin has been licensed for the treatment of cisplatin-induced anaemia during prolonged chemotherapy.

It can be seen that regular monitoring of the blood count is essential to allow changes in both the dose and scheduling of treatment to avoid severe myelotoxicity with all its complications. Prompt reduction in the dose of drugs, extension of the interval between courses of chemotherapy or the use of colony stimulating factors in appropriate cases, will usually prevent problems occurring. Extra care is needed in the presence of other clinical problems which affect the metabolism or excretion of a drug. For example, reduced renal function or marked ascites or pleural effusions, may increase the time that a cytotoxic drug (e.g. methotrexate) is retained in the body and therefore the exposure of the bone marrow to that drug, with resulting higher levels of marrow toxicity.

Nausea and vomiting, mucositis, and diarrhoea

Many cytotoxic drugs cause nausea and vomiting which can vary from mild to severe. Cisplatin is the most emetogenic of the cytotoxic agents used in treating gynaecological cancer. Emesis probably occurs because of the combination of stimuli from both the central nervous system and the bowel. The timing of the onset of symptoms can vary from shortly after injection, to 12 hours or more in the case of carboplatin, and their duration can be brief or persist for several days, as can occur with cisplatin. Prophylactic anti-emetic therapy with a phenothiazine or domperidone may be sufficient for some drug regimens that produce only mild symptoms, but for platinum regimens the most effective prophylactic antiemetic therapy is a combination of steroids and a 5-hydroxytryptamine (*serotonin*) ($5HT_3$)-receptor antagonist: either granisetron, ondansetron, or tropisetron. These are given intravenously prior to chemotherapy and orally afterwards (Table 10.2). Although the precise mode of action of $5HT_3$ antagonists is not known, they are thought to act on both the peripheral and central nervous system by preventing chemotherapy-induced $5HT$ release causing an effect at $5HT_3$ receptors. Reflexes from the small intestine are suppressed and the release of $5HT$ within the vomiting centre in the fourth ventricle of the brain, which occurs in response to these reflexes and as a direct effect of cytotoxic drugs, is reduced. Intravenous hydration may be necessary if vomiting leads to electrolyte disturbance.

Mouth ulcers, which occur most commonly with the antimetabolites, methotrexate and 5-flourouracil, are treated with mouth washes. With methotrexate, mucositis can be prevented by extending the period over which folinic acid rescue is given on subsequent courses of treatment. Ulceration may also affect the bowel mucosa causing diarrhoea and posing the threat of septicaemia. Intravenous hydration, electrolyte replacement, and drugs that slow bowel motility, such as codeine phosphate, are indicated in the management of this problem.

Renal tract toxicity

The nephrotoxicity of cisplatin, which is dose-related, leads to a fall in the glomerular filtration rate and tubular dysfunction. To reduce this complication, a high urine output is necessary. A diuresis of 100 ml urine per hour is maintained before, during and after administration of cisplatin by using

Table 10.6 Regimen for cisplatin therapy (50–75 mg/m^2)

Pre-hydration
1 litre normal saline plus 10 mmol MgSO$_4$, over 2 hours
1 litre normal saline plus 20 mmol KCl, over 2 hours
200 ml mannitol 20%, over 20 minutes (for forced diuresis prior to cisplatin)

Cisplatin
50–75 mg/m^2 in 1 litre normal saline, over 2 hours
Post-hydration
1 litre normal saline plus 10 mmol MgSO$_4$, over 2 hours
1 litre normal saline plus 20 mmol KCl, over 2 hours
The urine output should be maintained at more than 100 ml/hour

intravenous fluids and mannitol (Table 10.6). Glutathione, which has been found to have some nephro-protective properties, has been used with high dose cisplatin.

The drug dose must be reduced if renal function is shown to be impaired. Tests of renal function, such as EDTA or creatinine clearance tests, need to be performed before each course of cisplatin, as renal function can become cumulatively impaired during treatment. If the glomerular filtration rate falls to less than 50 ml per minute the drug should not be prescribed.

Methotrexate, given in high doses, can crystallize in the renal tubules causing renal damage. This can be avoided by ensuring that a high urine output is maintained throughout the period of drug administration and that the urine is kept alkaline by oral bicarbonate administration. This allows the drug to remain in solution in the urine and increases excretion. Both cyclophosphamide and ifosfamide produce metabolites that can act directly on the urothelium causing an haemorrhagic chemical cystitis. Acrolein, one of these metabolites, if present in large quantities, is the main cause of this chemical cystitis. This can be prevented by the use of high dose uromitexan (Mesna) which is given at the same time as the chemotherapy, and by maintaining a high fluid intake using an intravenous infusion. Uromitexan protects the urothelium by binding to acrolein in the urine thus making it inactive.

Alopecia

Alopecia is common after treatment with many drugs including the taxanes, cyclophosmide and ifosfamide, etoposide, and the antracyclines, such as doxorubicin. This is due to the high rate of turnover of the cells of the hair follicles. Usually, only the head hair is lost but with paclitaxel, all the body hair is affected. This hair loss is temporary and usually starts 3–4 weeks after commencing chemotherapy and can continue for up to 6 months following completion of chemotherapy. With the anthracyclines, because the drug is metabolized rapidly, hair loss can be much reduced by scalp cooling using special cold helmets which completely cover the hairline before and during administration of the drug. The scalp cooling causes vasospasm, reducing the amount of drug reaching the hair follicles. In cases where a wig is necessary careful counselling and the provision of the wig well in advance of hair loss helps to reduce the patient's anxiety.

Infertility and teratogenicity

Chemotherapy with alkylating agents, such as chlorambucil and cyclophosphamide, often causes infertility. However, successful pregnancies, producing normal children, have occurred in young women treated for germ cell tumours with combination cisplatin regimens. Menstruation may cease in perimenopausal women but there is usually only a temporary cessation in young women.

All cytotoxic chemotherapy must be considered to carry the risk of teratogenicity, which can continue after completion of drug therapy. Patients should be advised to avoid pregnancy during treatment and for at least one year after completing chemotherapy.

Neurotoxicity

Neurotoxicity most commonly occurs with paclitaxel, cisplatin, and vincristine. Peripheral sensory neuropathy and ototoxicity are the commonest complications of cisplatin. Central nervous system toxicity is rare because of an effective blood–brain barrier to cisplatin. Peripheral neuropathy is characterized by loss of tendon reflexes, paraesthesia, and numbness in a 'glove and stocking' distribution. This can lead to functional impairment if the cisplatin is not discontinued. Although the symptoms usually improve after cessation of the drug this can take months or years and may not be complete. This toxicity is directly related to cumulative dose rather than to the magnitude of each individual dose but scheduling plays a part, with neurological problems being more common with high dose therapy when the same dose is given over 5 days compared to two fractions 1 week apart. (Warner 1995).

Prevention of cisplatin peripheral neuropathy can be achieved by limiting the cumulative cisplatin dose, by using carboplatin in place of cisplatin whenever feasible because of its minimal neurotoxicity, and by the use of neuroprotective drugs. The use of these latter drugs is still largely experimental and include sulphur-containing compounds, such as WR-2721 (ethiofos) which is believed to inhibit directly interaction between cisplatin and peripheral nerves and which has been shown to reduce neuropathy when given with cisplatin. A neurotrophic drug, ORG 2766, an analogue of

ACTH, is thought to enhance recovery from nerve damage. Trials have shown equivocal results.

Ototoxicity, causing a high tone hearing loss and tinnitus with cisplatin, is related to many factors including dose per treatment, cumulative dose (greater than 170 mg/m^2), method of administration, pre-existing hearing loss, age, and renal function (Warner 1995). This ototoxicity may be due to an increase in cisplatin concentration in the 24 hours after the cessation of cisplatin therapy. No drugs have, as yet, been found to combat this problem.

Paclitaxel, particularly at high dose, can result in a variety of neurological problems. Those consist of a sensory and motor neuropathy as well as an autonomic neuropathy and myopathy. Previous treatment with other neurotoxic drugs, such as cisplatin, or diseases such as diabetes mellitus and chronic alcoholism, predispose patients to the development of neuropathies from paclitaxel. The most common neurological toxicity is peripheral neuropathy which frequently occurs with conventional doses, when it is usually mild. Peripheral neuropathy can start within 1–3 days after treatment with high doses but the effect is usually due to the cumulative dose. Mild symptoms usually resolve within months of stopping paclitaxel but severe symptoms can persist for more than one year. Motor neuropathy is rarely severe enough to cause clinical problems. Autonomic neuropathy, which can cause paralytic ileus and orthostatic hypotension, is rarely seen at doses below 250 mg/m^2, except in patients with diabetes mellitus. Myalgia, which affects the shoulder and paraspinal muscles, occurs with doses higher than 170 mg/m^2, 2–3 days after treatment and resolves within a few days.

The combination of paclitaxel and cisplatin at conventional dosage of 175 mg/m^2 for paclitaxel and 75 mg/m^2 for cisplatin does not appear to increase the risk of neurological toxicity. The neurotoxicity of paclitaxel appears to be attenuated when it is used with carboplatin.

Vincristine, as well as causing a peripheral neuropathy, may give rise to constipation and in extreme cases paralytic ileus due to an autonomic neuropathy. The development of paraesthesia or loss of tendon reflexes is treated by a dose reduction but if the symptoms becomes progressive the drug must be stopped.

High dose ifosfamide or cyclophosphamide can be toxic to the central nervous system (CNS) and can produce somnolence, hallucinations, and coma. This is rarely fatal and recovery is usually complete within a few days of stopping treatment. Methylene blue may be given intravenously to increase the rate of recovery from CNS toxicity or may be given prophylactically in patients who have suffered some CNA toxicity in previous courses. A nomogram that takes account of hepatic and renal function can produce an estimate of the likelihood of treatment causing central nervous system toxicity and, if a high risk is predicted, the drug should not be used.

Pulmonary toxicity

Bleomycin, cyclophosphamide, and methotrexate can all cause pulmonary changes which may be transient but may progress to pulmonary fibrosis. The dose reduction and other measures taken to prevent pulmonary fibrosis with bleomycin have been discussed (p. 214). Particular care must be taken in patients requiring general anaesthesia who have received bleomycin as they run a risk of respiratory failure if given high concentrations of oxygen.

Cardiotoxicity

Cardiomyopathy occurs with the anthracyclines. With doxorubicin, cardiomyopathy becomes a risk if the cumulative dose is greater than 450 mg/m^2, unless there has been previous radiotherapy to the chest when cardiotoxicity can occur at lower doses. Cardiac monitoring, for example by sequential radionuclide ejection fraction measurement (MUGA scan), should be carried out prior to and during a course of anthracyclines. The anthracyclines should not be given unless the patient's cardiac status is satisfactory and great care is needed in elderly patients in whom a dose reduction is recommended. Other drugs such as cyclophosphamide and 5-flourouracil can also be cardiotoxic, particularly after radiotherapy.

Liver damage

Serious liver damage is uncommon but can occur with the administration of methotrexate, particularly if it is given as a bolus. The damage can be either hepatic fibrosis that reverses on the cessation of treatment, or cirrhosis which is irreversible. Care must be taken when using this drug in patients with impaired hepatic function, in whom a reduction in dose in necessary.

Local damage at the injection site

Extravasation into tissues, when giving chemotherapy, can result in severe continuous pain, inflammation and, occasionally, tissue necrosis and ulceration. The anthracyclines, doxorubicin and epirubicin, cause a particularly severe reaction. Extravasation of vincristine can also result in significant tissue damage. Preventive measurements include giving such drugs in a fast-running drip and immediately stopping the infusion if there is any local pain. If extravasation occurs, the limb should be elevated and ice packs applied to the area. Injection of 1500 units of hyaluronidase subcutaneously can help disperse the drug and topical dimethyl sulphoxide has some effect in preventing local ulceration and scarring. The worst cases may need a skin graft. A plastic surgeon should supervize the management of all cases from the outset.

Drug resistance

Resistance to chemotherapy occurs when a tumour fails to respond or continues to grow during treatment (Fig. 10.6). In some gynaecological tumours there is little initial response due to *intrinsic* resistance to chemotherapy. In other tumours resistance is *acquired* and after an initial response, disease becomes resistant to the initial chemotherapy and often also to other cytotoxic agents. Both intrinsic and acquired resistance play an

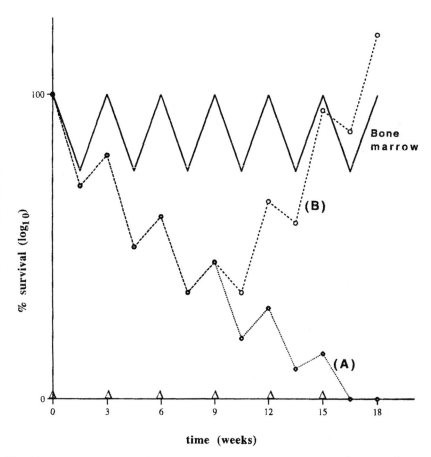

Fig. 10.6 Representation of the response of a tumour to treatment with cytotoxic chemotherapy. The 3-weekly treatment schedule allows for bone marrow regeneration between cycles (Δ shows the timing of each cycle of chemotherapy). (A) Successful treatment showing progressive reduction in tumour size until no clonogenic tumour cells remain. (B) Unsuccessful treatment where the growth kinetics of the tumour have changed at 9 weeks (e.g. because of acquisition of drug resistance).

important role in the response of gynaecological malignancies, notably ovarian cancer, to chemotherapy.

Tumour characteristics

There are multiple causes of chemoresistance. Some of these are due to characteristics of the tumour. For example, tumours which have a fast doubling time are more likely to be cured with chemotherapy than slow growing tumours. Some drugs, such as the antimetabolites and the anthracyclines act only on proliferating cells. Therefore, in *large tumours with a small growth fraction*, there tends to be a high degree of chemoresistance to such agents. However, with *small tumour burdens with a high growth fraction* (e.g. after surgery), there will be an increased response.

During growth, the cells within a tumour tend to accumulate a range of genetic mutations some of which confer a growth advantage. In addition, exposure to environmental 'stress', for instance in the form of cytotoxic chemotherapy, will tend to select out the resistant clones. This is the rationale for combination chemotherapy when, by using more than one drug, there should be an overall reduction in the risk of selecting drug-resistant clones. Drug resistance can also develop through the mechanism of *gene amplification* leading to the production of a protein which is able to maintain function despite the presence of a cytotoxic drug (Talbot and Philip 1995).

In large tumours, *poor vascularity* not only limits the amount of drug reaching the tumour but also results in *hypoxia* and hypoxic cells have been found to be chemoresistant as well as radioresistant. The exact nature of cellular resistance related to hypoxia is being researched but will be due, in some cases, to the need for metabolic activation of the cytotoxic drugs by enzyme systems which require oxygen. An example is the cytochrome P450 system in the liver which activates the oxazophosphorenes, cyclophosphamide, and ifosfamide.

Cellular mechanisms

Cellular mechanisms of resistance can be due to both biochemical and pharmacological mechanisms which lead to *a reduction in the intracellular concentration of a drug or drugs*. The drug can enter the cell by passive diffusion or by protein-mediated mechanisms. *Impaired membrane transport* has been shown to increase greatly resistance to drugs. For cisplatin, the drug gains access to the cell by both passive diffusion and by a gated facilitated diffusion channel (Gately and Howell 1993). Absence of this channel would result in partial drug resistance.

Exposure of tumour cells to one drug can lead to cross-resistance to other unrelated drugs to which the tumour has not been exposed. This phenomenon is known as *multi-drug resistance* (MDR). This occurs with drugs such as the anthracyclines, taxanes, podophyllotoxins, and the vinca alkaloids, and is due to changes in membrane permeability due to P-Gp, a 'permeability glycoprotein' which is an energy-dependent transporter pumping certain chemicals and hydrophobic drugs out of the cell, thereby stopping the cytotoxic drug's action on the cell. P-Gp is encoded by a group of closely related genes known as *mdr 1* which are on chromosome 7q21-1. Overexpression of these genes is found in the MDR phenotype. There are usually low levels of *mdr 1* and P-Gp expression in ovarian cancer indicating initial chemosensitivity.

Not all tumours that show multi-drug resistance overexpress P-Gp. MDR can be due to a multiplicity of genetic factors, one of which has been identified as a gene which encodes a protein termed *mrp* (multi-drug resistance-related protein) which is found in the endoplasmic reticulum as well as the plasma membrane.

Cell metabolism

Most cytotoxic drugs undergo bio-transformation in the liver but are then further metabolized by tumour cells (Talbot and Philip 1995). Drug resistance can be due to the action of enzymes within the cell concerned with detoxification, degradation, and metabolic activation. Reduced expression of the enzymes needed for the transformation of cyclophosphamide and ifosfamide to their active forms (e.g. by down-regulation in cancer cells of the cytochrome P-450-dependent mono-oxygenases), will lead to lower concentrations of the active chemicals.

Detoxification of drugs in cells is mainly carried out by cellular thiols, which include the tripeptide glutathione (GSH). Elevated levels of GSH are associated with increased drug resistance to cisplatin and other alkylating drugs and to the anthracyclines. Levels of glutathione S-transferases (GSTs), which are isoenzymes that act as catalysts for GSH-dependent detoxication reactions, tend to be raised in resistant cancer cells.

Cellular resistance to cytotoxic drugs may also arise from *alterations in nucleotide biosynthesis*, which protect the cancer cell from the inhibitory effect of cytotoxic drugs acting on essential enzymes necessary for the synthesis and maintenance of DNA. One example is reduction in tumour cell levels of topisomerase II, one of two classes of topoisomerases which are nuclear enzymes essential in DNA transcription and replication. This reduction leads to resistance to drugs which act by inhibiting topoisomerase II (e.g. etoposide).

The ability of a cell to *repair* the damage caused by cytotoxic drugs will also affect cell resistance as most cytotoxcic agents act by directly or indirectly damaging DNA. Increased repair will lead to increased resistance.

Despite increasing knowledge in regard to the mechanisms underlying drug resistance, it is still unknown why some tumours are inherently resistant to chemotherapeutic agents. It is thought that this may be related, at least in part, to the genes that control apoptosis (programmed cell death). The genes involved include *bcl-2*, which inhibits drug-induced apoptosis, *myc* and *P53*. Alterations in the expression of these genes may well provide a common pathway for resistance to a range of different cytotoxic drugs by means of inhibition of drug-induced apoptosis. Further research in this area may well hold the key to dealing with drug resistance.

Methods to reduce drug resistance

The clinical methods to overcome drug resistance are summarized in Table 10.7. The main clinical methods are a high cytotoxic dose intensity to overcome intrinsic resistance, combination chemotherapy using drugs with different cellular actions, alternating non-cross-resistant chemotherapy or alternative scheduling (e.g. by continuous infusion of 5FU). Drugs are being developed to block multi-drug resistance (MDR). These drugs act by binding with P-Gp. Some of these drugs are calcium channel blockers, such as verapamil and nifedipine. Other MDR inhibitors include the anti-

Table 10.7 Methods to overcome cell resistance to chemotherapy

Clinical	
1. Overcoming cytokinetic resistance	• Increased dose intensity
	• Combination chemotherapy
	• Alternating chemotherapy (non-cross-resistant)
	• Schedule-guided treatment
2. Reducing host toxicity	• Altering route of administration
	• Normal tissue rescue
	• Haemopoeitic growth factors
	• Peripheral stem cell rescue
Experimental	
3. Biochemical modulation	• Inhibitors of multi-drug resistance
	• Hypoxically activated drugs
	• Inhibitors of DNA repair enzymes
	• Inhibitors of drug detoxification
	• Analogues with greater cellular retention
4. Novel approaches	• Antibody-directed enzyme-pro-drug therapy (ADEPT)
	• Gene-directed enzyme-pro-drug-therapy (GDEPT)
	• Modulation of tumour oncogene expression
	• Inhibition of signal transduction pathways
	• Gene therapy

Modified from Talbot and Philip (1995).

oestrogen tamoxifen but as the doses needed to inhibit P-Gp cause severe neurotoxicity, similar drugs, such as toremifene are being investigated. At present these approaches have not been successful *in vivo* because of unacceptable toxicity.

Conclusions

The curative role of chemotherapy in gynaecological cancer is limited to the treatment of germ cell and trophoblastic tumours.

Adjuvant chemotherapy in ovarian cancer has led to a prolongation of median survival and disease-free survival but not five-year overall survival. Neo-adjuvant chemotherapy is being studied in the management of advanced cervical and vulvar cancer.

Drug resistance remains the most serious problem in the use of chemotherapy as a treatment modality with curative intent.

Because of the toxicity of chemotherapy, and the need for expertise in the management of life-threatening complications resulting from such therapy, chemotherapy should only be given under the supervision of specialists who have been trained in the use of cytotoxic drugs.

References

Alberts, D. S., Liu, P. Y., Hannigan, E. V. *et al.* (1996). Intraperitoneal cisplatin plus intravenous cyclophosphamide versus intravenous cisplatin plus intravenous cyclophosphamide for stage III ovarian cancer. *New England Journal of Medicine*, 335, 1950–5.

Calvert, A. H., Newell, D. R., Gumbrell, L. A. *et al.* (1987). Carboplatin dosage: Prospective evaluation of a simple formula based on renal function. *Journal of Clinical Oncology*, 7, 1748–56.

Cockroft, D. W. and Gault, M. H. (1976). Prediction of creatinine clearance from serum creatinine. *Nephron*, 16, 31–41.

Gately, D. P. and Howell, S. B. (1993). Cellular accumulation of the anticancer agent cisplatin: a review. *British Journal of Cancer*, 67, 1171.

Gelmon, K. (1994). The taxoids: paclitaxel and docetaxel. *Lancet*, 344, 1267–71.

Goldie, J. H. and Coldman, A. J. (1979). A mathematical model for relating the drug sensitivity of tumours to their spontaneous mutation rate. *Cancer Treatment Report*, 63, 1727–33.

Lambert, H. E., Rustin, J. S., Gregory, W. M., Nelstrop, A. E. (1997). A randomised trial of 5 versus 8 courses of cisplatin or carboplatin in advanced epithelial ovarian cancer (a North Thames Ovary Group study). *Annals of Oncology*, 8, 327–33.

Norton, L. and Simon, R. (1977). Tumour size, sensitivity to therapy and design of treatment schedules. *Cancer Treatment Report*, 61, 1307–17.

Skipper, H.E., Schabel, F. H., Wilcox, W. S. *et al.* (1964). Experimental evaluation of potential anticancer agents. XIII: on the criteria and kinetics associated with availability of experimental leukaemia. *Cancer Chemotherapy Report*, 35, 1–11.

Slevin, M. L., Clark, P. I., Joel, S. P. *et al.* (1989). A randomized trial to evaluate the effect of schedule on the activity of etoposide in small cell lung cancer. *Journal of Clinical Oncology*, 7, 1333–40.

Steward, W. P., Cassidy, J., and Kaye, S. B. (1995). Principles of chemotherapy. In *Treatment of cancer* (3rd edn) (ed. P. Price and K. Sikora), pp. 91–108. Chapman and Hall, London.

Talbot, D. C. and Philip, P. A. (1995). Drug resistance. In *Treatment of cancer* (3rd end) (ed. P. Price and K. Sikora), pp. 109–20. Chapman and Hall, London.

ten Bookkel Huinink, W. W., Eisenhauer, E., and Swenerton, K. (1993). For the Canadian–European Taxol Cooperative Trial Group. Preliminary evaluation of a multicentre, randomised comparative study of taxol (paclitaxel) dose and infusion length in platinum-treated ovarian cancer. *Cancer Treatment Review*, **19** (Suppl.C), 79–86.

Warner, E. (1995). Neurotoxicity of cisplatin and taxol. *International Journal of Gynecological Cancer*, 5, 161.

11

Palliation of gynaecological malignancy

Introduction

Despite recent advances in treatment, at least 50 percent of women diagnosed with gynaecological cancer will die of the disease. Therefore, the need to palliate the distressing symptoms associated with advanced malignancy is very important.

Palliative care is best described as the active total care of a person whose disease is no longer responsive to curative treatment. This encompasses pain and symptom control and emphasizes the importance of psychological, social, and spiritual issues. The goal of palliative care is to achieve the best quality of life for the patient and their family or carers (WHO 1990). Ideally, palliative care should be available throughout the disease process and not just in the terminal phase.

Although some of the common symptoms of gynaecological malignancy may be due to treatment, more often they occur as a result of disease progression. If further anti-cancer treatment is available then it is the most effective method of palliation. The potential benefits should be weighed up against the probable adverse effects, and this information should be discussed with the patient and her family before embarking upon treatment.

The main causes of symptoms in advanced gynaecological cancer are:

1. Local disease within the pelvis or abdomen causing infiltration, pressure or ulceration.

2. Distant spread with metastases in the liver, lung, bone, or brain.

3. Treatment with chemotherapy, radiotherapy, or medication.

4. Incidental cause such as infection or coexisting illness.

Symptom control may be achieved by treating the cancer with surgery, radiotherapy, or chemotherapy. Where these measures fail or are inappropriate other symptom-specific measures need to be used. This chapter addresses some of the more common symptoms and their management.

Pain

Pain has been defined as 'an unpleasant sensory and emotional experience associated with actual or potential tissue damage or described in terms of such damage' (IASP 1986). Although it is a common misconception that pain is inevitable with cancer, it is known that between 20–50% of patients have pain at the time of presentation. The prevalence of this increases to 75% in those patients with advanced cancer.

Many myths surround cancer pain and its management. There is a widely held belief among patients (and indeed doctors) that analgesic drugs, in particular morphine, are addictive and should therefore be reserved for when a patient is about to die. This myth persists resulting in a 'phobia' about morphine. A further hindrance to good pain management is the reluctance of patients to take medications. Some patients stop medication when they develop side-effects without realizing that these can be avoided or corrected, or that alternative analgesic agents are available.

Evaluation

Careful assessment and evaluation is essential for successful pain control. It is of primary importance to establish a cause by taking a complete pain history (Table 11.1). The patient's own description of the pain can help with this (Table 11.2). It should be remembered that some patients may be too frightened to mention pain or may minimize their symptoms as it implies spread or recurrence of disease. Additional information may be gained by discussion with family or carers. There are many validated pain assessment tools such as the Wisconsin Brief Pain Inventory and the McGill Pain Questionnaire which can be helpful. Commonly, patients have more than one pain and a body chart can be useful for identifying the different sites. The cause may be obvious after history and examination but investigations may be required.

Table 11.1 Essential elements of the pain history

- Site
- Quality and description of the pain
- Exacerbating/relieving factors
- Onset of pain
- Associated symptoms (insomnia, depression)
- How the pain interferes with everyday life
- Psychological state of the patient
- Response to current and previous pain therapies

Table 11.2 Common causes and descriptions of pain in malignancy

Source of pain	Typical description of pain
Visceral infiltration	
Stretching of fascia	Dull ache
Obstruction of hollow viscus	Colicky or cramping
Bone metastases	Dull, constant ache
	Often exacerbated by movement
Nerve infiltration or compression	Continuous ache
	Burning
	Intermittent stabbing pain (associated with an area of abnormal or absent sensation)

General management

Once established, the cause of the pain should be explained to the patient. Analgesia should be initiated immediately without waiting for the results of tests. Doctors often fail in pain relief because they describe drugs in-appropriately, without thinking of the likely cause of the pain and without adequate explanation of their use. By adhering to the simple guidelines recommended by the World Health Organisation (WHO), pain can be controlled in 80–90% of cases (WHO 1986).

The WHO analgesic ladder

The WHO analgesic ladder is a well-established approach to the manage-ment of cancer pain (Fig. 11.1). This approach advocates analgesic medication being administered regularly and preferably by the oral route—constant pain requires regular analgesia. There are three steps to the ladder and if pain persists then a move to the next step is required, rather than the prescribing of an alternative drug of the same efficacy. At each step of the ladder, adjuvant analgesic drugs may be added when necessary. These drugs

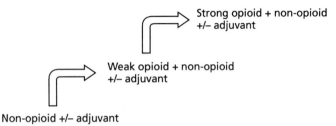

Strong opioid + non-opioid +/– adjuvant

Weak opioid + non-opioid +/– adjuvant

Non-opioid +/– adjuvant

Fig. 11.1 The World Health Organization three-step analgesic ladder (WHO 1986).

are primarily used for indications other than pain but are effective analgesic drugs in some conditions.

Step 1 includes non-opioid drugs, such as paracetamol and aspirin, with paracetamol being more commonly prescribed in the UK. These are used for mild to moderate pain. The non-steroidal anti-inflammatory drugs (NSAIDs) can also be included at this step. NSAIDs have a specific analgesic effect as well as acting to reduce pain by modifying the inflammatory process. The non-opioid drugs may be beneficial when used in conjunction with the drugs at higher steps in the ladder.

Step 2 represents the weak opioid drugs, with the most commonly used being codeine, dihydrocodeine, and dextropropoxyphene. These should be given regularly and to their maximal dose before a move in the next step is considered. Dihydrocodeine has the advantage of being available in a slow-release preparation which can be given twice daily. Some combination preparations of weak opioid drugs contain subtherapeutic doses of one or both constituents and should be avoided. However, coproxamol does contain therapeutic doses of both paracetamol and dextropropoyxphene and may be useful. Tramadol hydrochloride is a centrally acting analgesic drug which acts at opioid receptors. The analgesic effect may be enhanced by its action of increasing serotonin release and inhibiting re-uptake of noradrenaline in the dorsal horn cells. It is useful in mild to moderate pain. It does not fit in neatly to the WHO ladder and should considered between *step* 2 and *step* 3. It is thought to cause less constipation and sedation than morphine.

Step 3, although there are other opioids available, morphine remains the WHO strong opioid of choice at this step of the analgesic ladder.

Morphine

Oral morphine is available in several preparations (Table 11.3). Immediate release (IR) morphine is the most effective for establishing a patient's opioid requirement rapidly. It has an onset of action of 20 minutes to 1 hour and the analgesic activity lasts for 4 hours. The typical starting dose when changing from a weak opioid would be 10 mg every 4 hours. To avoid disturbing the patient's sleep, it is common practice to administer a 'double-dose' (i.e. twice the 4-hourly dose) at night. The 4-hourly dose of morphine should also be prescribed, to be taken as required, for 'breakthrough' pain. A patient should never be expected to wait for analgesia if they are in pain and 'breakthrough' doses can be given as often as needed. Pain should be reassessed regularly as the need for multiple doses of 'breakthrough' may indicate the need to increase the basic 4-hourly dose of morphine. If pain control has not been achieved, morphine doses can be increased every 24 hours. There is no ceiling dose for morphine as the correct dose is that

Table 11.3 Oral preparation of morphine

Duration of action	4 hours (immediate release)	12 hours (delayed release)	24 hours (delayed release)
Tablet	Sevredol (mg); 10, 20, 50	MST Continus or Oramorph SR (mg): 5, 10, 13, 30, 60, 100, 200	
Capsule (can be broken open)			MXL (mg): 30, 60, 90, 120, 180
Solution	Oramorph liquid (mg/5 ml): 10, 100 Oramorph unit dose vials (mg/5 ml): 10, 30, 100		
Suspension		MST Continus (mg): 20, 30, 60, 100, 200	

which controls the patients pain. It should be noted that not all pain is morphine-responsive, especially neuropathic pain and bone pain. Although morphine may be beneficial, an adjuvant analgesic may be necessary.

A stable dose of morphine is one which controls pain for two days with only two breakthrough doses of morphine in twenty four hours. At this point the patient can be converted to one of the slow-release preparations of morphine. The total dose of morphine taken in 24 hours is calculated and given as either a once daily capsule or divided into two doses using sustained release tablets or suspension. Slow-release forms of morphine maintain the serum morphine levels at a steady state and can improve patient compliance.

Morphine is metabolized in the liver and is renally excreted together with the metabolites. The major metabolites are morphine-6-glucuronide (which also has analgesic activity) and morphine-3-glucuronide. If renal function is compromised, morphine and the metabolites will accumulate resulting in toxicity. This may present as confusion, drowsiness, and myoclonic jerking. Morphine may still be used but the dose will need to reduced and the dose interval increased.

Constipation is an inevitable side-effect of morphine and therefore, unless the patient has diarrhoea, laxatives should always be prescribed prophylactically. The laxatives prescribed should work by softening stool (e.g. docusate sodium) and should help to stimulate bowel peristalsis (e.g. senna). Bulk-forming laxatives should be avoided. Nausea and vomiting may occur during the first few days of starting morphine and the patient should be prescribed anti-emetic medication as a precaution (haloperidol 1.5 mg at night is commonly used). In most instances nausea resolves within two or three days but in a few cases long-term anti-emetic cover is necessary. Many patients taking morphine complain of a dry mouth and this particular problem often persists. Other side-effects are drowsiness, which tends to wear off after a few days, and occasionally pruritus and confusion. If the latter two problems persist it is usual to change to an alternate opioid.

When a patient cannot manage to take analgesia by mouth, because of dysphagia, nausea, or vomiting, decreased level of consciousness or because they are too weak to swallow, a different route must be considered. Morphine can be given rectally or parenterally. Where parenteral administration is required in the UK, diamorphine tends to be used rather than morphine as it is far more soluble and is easily mixed with anti-emetics and other drugs. It can be given subcutaneously (sc) either via an indwelling butterfly needle as a regular bolus or preferably by a continuous syringe driver infusion. The relative potency of sc diamorphine to oral morphine is 1:3 (10 mg sc diamorphine is equivalent to 30 mg of oral morphine) (Twycross 1994).

Alternate opioids

Alternate opioids are available for sublingual, rectal, subcutaneous, and transdermal delivery. The most commonly used alternate opioids with the route of administration are listed (Table 11.4). The indications for using an alternate opioid are where there are persistent unacceptable side-effects with morphine, when analgesia administered by an alternative route may

Table 11.4 Alternate opioids

Drug	Preparation	Indication	Comment
Diamorphine	Injection	Parenteral opioid required	More soluble than morphine
Phenazocine	Tablets	Intolerance to morphine	5 mg tablets only, can be used sublingually
Fentanyl	Transdermal patch	Intolerance to morphine, poor compliance, alternate route of delivery required	Not suitable for rapidly changing analgesic requirements
Methadone	Liquid, tablets and injection	Intolerance to morphine, possibly a specific role in neuropathic pain	Long half-life; *beware* of toxic metabolic accumulation
Oxycodone	Tablets and suppositories	Intolerance to morphine, alternate route of delivery required	Useful for headache due to raised intracranial pressure
Hydromorphone	Tablets and injection	Intolerance to morphine	Widely used in North America
Dextromoramide	Tablets and suppositories	Incident pain (e.g. prior to dressing changes)	Short duration of action, not useful for chronic pain
Pethidine	Tablets and injection	*Not* indicated for chronic pain	Short duration of action, tablets poorly absorbed Accumulation of toxic metabolites with regular use

improve compliance (e.g. transdermal) or will be more effective (e.g. use of the rectal or subcutaneous route when a patient is vomiting). In some cases an alternate opioid is given because of morphine phobia (doctor or patient phobia).

Specific pain management

Neuropathic pain

Neuropathic pain (Table 11.2) is due to peripheral or central nerve damage or pressure. Although opioids may partly relieve the pain, adjuvant drugs are commonly required. Tricyclic antidepressants, anticonvulsants, and the oral local anaesthetic drugs are frequently used in such cases (Portenoy 1993). These and other drugs that have been used in neuropathic pain are listed in Table 11.5.

Antidepressants, such as amitriptyline and dothiepin, are typically used for 'aching' or 'burning' pain and are started at a low dose at night which is then increased slowly over a period of days. The onset of action is faster

Table 11.5 Commonly used adjuvant analgesic drugs

Pain	Drug category	Examples	Typical doses
Bone pain	Biphosphonate	Pamidronate disodium, clodronate	Variable: awaiting results of doses and frequency from trials
	Corticosteroid	Dexamethasone, prednisolone	Dexamethasone 4–8 mg per day
Neuropathic	Tricyclic antidepressant	Amitritriptyline, dothiepin	Low starting dose: initially 10 mg in the elderly; 25 mg in general. Effective dose varies from 50 to 150 mg at night
	Anticonvulsant	Sodium valproate, carbamazepine	Initially 100 mg twice daily to be increased slowly
	Oral local anaesthetic	Mexilitine, flecainide	Flecainide 100–200 mg twice daily, mexilitine 150 mg twice or thrice daily
	Corticosteroid	Dexamethasone, prednisolone	Up to 16 mg of dexamethasone per day
	Calcium antagonist	Nifedepine, diltiazem	Variable
	Miscellaneous	Baclofen	Variable
Smooth muscle spasm	Calcium antagonist Anticholinergic	Nifedepine, diltiazem Hyoscine butyl- or hydrobromide	Variable
Skeletal muscle spasm	Benzodiazepine Miscellaneous	Diazepam, lorazepam Baclofen	Diazepam 2–5 mg twice daily Variable

than that reported for treatment of depression with responses seen at about 10 days. The mode of action is thought to involve an increase in the levels of serotonin and noradrenaline in the brainstem and dorsal horn cells. These chemicals are involved in the inhibitory pain pathways. The side-effects of antidepressants include sedation, dry mouth, and orthostatic hypotension which limit their use. Cardiotoxicity can occur but is rare.

Anticonvulsants, such as sodium valproate and carbamazepine, are commonly used for stabbing pain. These drugs are thought to exert their effects by inhibiting spontaneous discharge from nerves. Again, they are started at low dose which is increased over a few days. The onset of response varies, being 3–5 days. The dose is empirical but may be a lower dose than that required for control of epilepsy. Side-effects include sedation, dizziness, and nausea. Both groups of drugs can be combined and may increase the effectiveness of opioids.

When the above drugs fail or the side-effects prohibit their use, the oral local anaesthetics, flecainide and mexilitine, could be considered (Portenoy 1993). The onset of action is about three days and although the drugs block sodium channels they may also suppress aberrant electrical activity in damaged nerves. The most common side-effects are nausea, vomiting, and dizziness. Flecainide should be used with caution when there is a previous cardiac history and avoided where there is evidence of atrioventricular block.

Bone pain

Bone pain can occur as a result of local disease spread within the pelvis or paravertebral region or from bone metastases. For specific areas of bone pain, radiotherapy, given as either a single fraction or as a course, can be extremely effective. Analgesia is usually required in addition to radio-therapy, especially if there is more general bone pain. Opioids may be effective alone but the addition of a NSAID may be required. If a patho-logical fracture or substantial loss of cortex of bone has occurred in a long bone then surgical fixation should be considered.

Bisphosphonates, potent inhibitors of osteoclast-mediated bone resorption, have also been used in the treatment of bone pain but further studies to determine dosages and dose schedules are awaited (Ernst *et al.* 1992).

Specific pain syndromes in gynaecological malignancy

Pelvic pain

Pelvic pain may be described as a dull, dragging pain referred to the lower back. This results from pressure due to localized tumour. Where there is adherence of the tumour to the pelvic side wall, the pain can be aggravated by walking. Often a combination of strong opioids and NSAIDs are required for effective pain management.

Lumbosacral plexopathy

This syndrome consists of sacral, buttock and leg pain often with associated limb weakness and lymphoedema. It may be seen in conjunction with hydronephrosis. The most frequent cause is prevertebral recurrence or extension of disease, although in rare cases radiation fibrosis may present with pain. The pain may be due to a combination of soft tissue invasion, nerve infiltration, and bone involvement. If there is disease in the lumbar region, infiltration of the psoas muscle can cause pain on hip extension. When possible, radiotherapy is an effective means of pain control used in conjunction with opioids and NSAIDs. There is often a need for adjuvant analgesics for the neuropathic component of pain. If pain is difficult to control by these means anaesthetic techniques using spinally administered drugs, such as epidural morphine and local anaesthetic, are effective.

Tenesmus

Tenesmus is a sensation of rectal fullness with a desire to evacuate. It can be associated with shooting pains in the rectum and may be aggravated by sitting or defaecating. It can be due to tumour invasion of the rectal wall or from involvement of the sacral plexus. The pain can respond to opioids but frequently requires adjuvant medication for neuropathic pain. Anticonvulsants have been found to be effective, as have calcium antagonists (Castell 1985). Locally applied steroids, in the form of enemas or foam, or NSAIDs (given orally or rectally) have also been tried. If the symptoms fail to respond adequately it is worth considering a sympathetic nerve block which has been reported as being extremely successful (Bristow and Foster 1988).

Perineal pain

Perineal pain may be a generalized ache together with shooting or burning pain in the perineum. Patients sometimes complain that they feel as if they are sitting on a lump. The pain may be brought on by sitting and, when severe, patients avoid this and either lie or stand. The pain is due to local recurrence involving the perineal nerves and usually responds to opioid drugs together with an adjuvant analgesic for the neuropathic element, occasionally with a NSAID. Where these measures fail, epidurally administered local anaesthetics or intrathecal drugs can be effective.

Nausea and vomiting

Nausea and vomiting occur in up to 50 percent of patients with advanced cancer, frequently together, but sometimes in isolation. Although nausea

Table 11.6 Causes of nausea and vomiting

Metabolic
- hypercalcaemia
- uraemia

Raised intracranial pressure: cerebral metastases

Drug-induced

Chemotherapy

Radiotherapy

Gastrointestinal cause
- constipation
- gastric distension and stasis
- bowel obstruction

Pain

Anxiety

and vomiting are generally multi-factorial, there are commonly identifiable causes (Table 11.6). If a particular cause is thought to be reversible, it should be treated specifically. Frequently, however, this is not possible and anti-emetics are required.

There are a large number of anti-emetics available, with different mechanisms of action and different uses (Table 11.7). Although in most cases the oral route is preferred, if intractable vomiting prevents this, other routes must be considered. These include sublingual, rectal, subcutaneous, and intravenous administration. A subcutaneous infusion or regular sub-cutaneous injections can be the most useful, particularly so in the treatment of bowel obstruction. Most of the commonly used drugs can be combined in a syringe driver with morphine or diamorphine. Once symptoms improve, patients should be converted back onto an oral preparation.

Bowel obstruction

Bowel obstruction is a common event in advanced gynaecological malignancy, in particular in ovarian cancer. The symptoms of nausea, vomiting, abdominal distension, constipation, and colicky abdominal pain tend to present insidiously, but can also present as an acute episode. In some cases, the bowel obstruction can be intermittent, where symptoms settle without intervention, but more often it will persist.

Surgical management

The prognosis for patients with malignant bowel obstruction is generally poor. Although rarely appropriate in advanced disease, palliative surgery

Table 11.7 Commonly used anti-emetic drugs, their route of administration and uses

Drug	Usual dose and route of administration	Typical dose in 24 h sc infusion	Specific uses, apart from general anti-emetic
Cyclizine	50 mg tds: po, sc, iv	150 mg over 24 h	Bowel obstruction, vertigo
Haloperidol	1.5–3 mg od or bd: po, sc, iv	3–10 mg over 24 h	Opioid induced nausea, bowel obstruction, and uraemia
Domperidone	10–20 mg: po; 30–60 mg: pr: tds or qds	Not available	Gastric stasis
Metoclopramide	10 mg tds: po, sc, iv	30 mg over 24 h	Gastric stasis
Prochlorperazine	5–10 mg tds: po 3–6 mg bd: buccal 5 mg tds; 25 mg stat-pr	Not suitable	Vertigo
Methotrimeprazine	6.25–12.5 mg od or bd: po or sc	25–150 mg over 24 h	Bowel obstruction and where sedation is required
Hyoscine	200–400 mcg tds: sc 500 mcg transdermal —lasts 3 days	800–1200 mcg over 24 h	Bowel obstruction where cramping is also a problem
Ondansetron	4–8 mg: bd po or iv	Has been used as a continuous infusion: 8 mg	Chemotherapy-induced nausea, bowel obstruction, and nausea due to uraemia
Granisetron	1 mg bd: po 3 mg: iv	Not known	Chemotherapy-induced nausea
Dexamethasone	4–16 mg od: po, iv, sc	4–16 mg (tends to precipitate when mixed with other drugs at high doses)	Raised incracranial pressure, liver metastases

Abbreviations: po, by mouth; sc, subcutaneous; iv, intravenous; pr, anally; od, once daily; bd, twice daily; tds, three times a day; qds, four times a day.

should always be considered. Patients with limited disease who are thought to have one point of obstruction may benefit from a palliative procedure, especially where further anti-cancer treatments are an option. Otherwise, the effectiveness of surgery is a contentious issue. Invariably the success of surgery has been measured in terms of survival, but this can be as short as two to three months and recurrence of obstruction can occur. Quality of life during and after surgery is rarely addressed and yet surgical procedures in women with advanced gynaecological malignancy carry a high rate of mortality and morbidity. Complications are common and include infection, leakage of bowel contents, and the formation of fistulae. Surgery is generally contraindicated in women who have multiple partial occlusions of the bowel or diffuse abdominal disease, ascites, low albumen, or who have had previous radiotherapy.

Medical management

Conservative management of bowel obstruction addresses the symptoms of nausea, vomiting, and pain. Parenteral anti-emetics, as discussed earlier, should be administered regularly or continuously (low dose metoclopramide and all other pro-kinetic anti-emetics are best avoided as they may aggravate colic). The pain of bowel obstruction, a dull ache or feeling of pressure, combined with intermittent colicky pain, will generally respond to diamorphine with possibly the addition of hyoscine-butyl-bromide for severe colic. Analgesics and anti-emetics may be combined together and given via a syringe driver. Initially, the bowel is rested and fluid replacement is given intravenously. The use of a nasogastric tube is common hospital practice especially where there is high-output vomiting.

With the above measures the obstruction may settle. The addition of high dose parenteral steroids together with suppositories or enemas, when constipation may have aggravated the conditions, can be of benefit. The role and effectiveness of steroids has never been proven but they possibly help resolution by reducing oedema and inflammation associated with the obstruction. Once obstruction has resolved, the risk of recurrence may be reduced by a low fibre diet and regular gentle laxatives. Stimulant laxatives may aggravate colic and should be avoided. Overall, however, the symptoms frequently recur within weeks.

When bowel obstruction does not resolve or where it is felt to be a terminal event at presentation, it is possible to keep symptoms well controlled until death. Vomiting can be managed using the above measures without a nasogastric tube (Baines *et al.* 1985). Placement of the tube may be distressing, and its presence irritating or upsetting. Patients may prefer to have an occasional vomit to having a nasogastric tube passed. The only time a nasogastric tube may be of great benefit is where there is a high level of obstruction resulting in frequent large vomits. An alternative may be insertion of a gastrostomy tube to drain the stomach contents (Ashby *et al.* 1991). This can be placed either during endoscopy or using ultrasound guidance. Both of these measures will allow the patient to eat and drink freely. These procedures may be avoided through the use of octreotide. This is an analogue of somatostatin that is becoming more widely used when there is frequent troublesome vomiting associated with obstruction. Octreotide is an inhibitory peptide which decreases intestinal secretion and promotes fluid and electrolyte absorption from the bowel. It also has the effect of decreasing peristalsis, thereby reducing colic. It has led to improved symptom management and quality of life in many patients (Mercadente *et al.*

1993). Octreotide can be given subcutaneously by bolus or by continuous infusion, initially at a dose of 300 µg in 24 hours, with few side-effects. Patients should be allowed to eat and drink as they wish.

Parenteral fluids are not always required in the long term. In fact, the use of intravenous fluids when a patient is dying may reduce close contact with the family and may preclude the opportunity for them to be at home. Where vomiting is controlled, frequent sips of fluid may relieve a dry mouth. The dry mouth is often caused by the drugs being used to control symptoms and this is best managed by local measures. If parenteral fluid is thought to be essential for symptom control it may be administered by hyperdermoclysis (sc) as an infusion (Fainsinger *et al.* 1994), or in intermittent bolus (Bruera *et al.* 1995, thus avoiding the need for painful cannulae insertion. This can often be managed at home.

Haemorrhage

Haemorrhage can occur in all gynaecological malignancies, but is more common in cervical and endometrial cancer. Bleeding may have been the patient's presenting symptom and therefore the return of this symptom can be distressing and frightening. Explanation and reassurance may enable a women to live with bleeding when it is mild, however, it is likely that the loss will increase progressively. Treatment options should be discussed, or at least considered at the outset. If patients are prescribed aspirin or anticoagulation therapy for previous deep-vein thrombosis this should be discontinued, the emphasis being on symptom control rather than prevention of other problems.

Sudden heavy blood loss can be halted by vaginal packing but can frequently recur once the packs are removed. If the packs are soaked in tranexamic acid prior to packing the haemostatic effect may be prolonged but this is only a temporary measure and is not for long-term use. If the bleeding is most likely to be a terminal event, the patient should be kept comfortable. Analgesia, as described before, and anxiolytics such as midazolam should be prescribed.

For more long-term bleeding, radiotherapy, either external beam or brachytherapy, can bring about control rapidly, but may not be an option if the patient has had extensive prior treatment. In this situation use of an antifibrinolytic agent, such as tranexamic acid, given orally can reduce the bleeding. Historically, ligation of the internal iliac arteries was a treatment for haemorrhage. There is now the option of embolization of pelvic bleeding. In patients where it is appropriate, angiography can define the blood supply of the tumour and embolization can be performed with either small gelfoam particles or coils. As a result, blood loss can be reduced or stopped, and pain control improved due the subsequent reduction in tumour size. Survival may be many months (Hendrickx *et al.* 1995). This procedure is gaining in popularity and has been successfully used for bleeding due to benign or malignant causes.

Vaginal discharge

Pelvic tumours will often result in vaginal discharge. If radiotherapy is still an option it can reduce secretions. Often, the discharge is due to necrotic tumour which has already received maximal radiotherapy. The aim of treatment should be to reduce discharge and its associated problems. Offensive odour is often the biggest problem for a patient and can lead to social and sexual isolation. If infection is thought to be the cause of worsening offensive discharge, a course of antibiotics should be prescribed. As the causative organisms are frequently anaerobes, metronidazole is the drug of choice. If symptoms fail to improve, antibiotics should be discontinued as they may cause or exacerbate nausea. The use of topical metronidazole gel directly into the vagina may be helpful in reducing odour, but it is unlikely to eradicate infection. The use of deodorizers or aromatherapy oils on a pad can also be considered but often the underlying odour remains. Vaginal pessaries such as povidone iodine have only a limited use as they tend to irritate normal vaginal tissue and can cause skin reactions. Although they may be difficult to introduce due to distortion of the pelvic anatomy, tampons may be helpful for absorbing discharge thereby allowing a more normal lifestyle. There is a risk of bleeding when anything is introduced into the vagina where there is necrotic tumour.

Fistulae

Ideal management of a fistula is surgical excision and repair, or diversion using a colostomy or ileal conduit. However, when caused by progressive and advanced cancer, with or without radiation damage, curative surgery is rarely an option. Care is focused on addressing the symptoms and supporting the patient. This may involve reducing or containing the fluid leak and protecting the surrounding skin. Again, offensive odour may be a major problem leading to isolation.

Enterovaginal fistulae

The discharge from a fistula between the terminal ileum and vagina tends to be yellowish and watery. The content is extremely alkaline and contains digestive enzymes so that surrounding skin becomes excoriated with resultant severe pain. Patients with sigmoid or rectovaginal fistulae pass brownish discharge, often with lumps of hard faeces. Although this can be acidic, there is less skin inflammation and pain.

It is difficult to contain leakage from the vagina so the skin should be protected using barrier creams. Local anaesthetic cream or barrier cream mixed with lignocaine can be soothing and, more recently, a thermo-reversible gel containing lignocaine has been used successfully and is currently undergoing further trials (MacGregor *et al.* 1994). If the skin is intact, it can be covered by a semi-occlusive dressing. Regular cleansing of the perineum is necessary together with regular changing of absorbent pads. A tampon, acting as plug and continence aid, can be used for short periods of time where the discharge is non-irritant.

Varying the consistency of the stool may, on occasion, reduce the output from the fistula. In small bowel fistulae this may be achieved by solidifying bowel contents using loperamide, codeine phosphate, or bulk-forming laxatives, such as ispaghula husk. In some cases the development of a fistula represents the resolution of bowel obstruction and, therefore, treatment of the fistula can result in recurrence of obstruction and is best avoided. Leakage from a large bowel fistula may be aggravated by constipation and may be reduced if this is addressed. If laxatives are prescribed it is important to avoid those containing danthron which can burn the skin.

Secretion from the bowel can sometimes be reduced by using octreotide. This may reduce the output of fluid from the small bowel, occasionally from the large bowel and may help to promote absorption (Nubiola-Calonge *et al.* 1987). Thus the loss from the fistula may be reduced. If octreotide fails to work within a few days it should be stopped.

Enterocutaneous fistulae

The measures above also apply to the treatment of enterocutaneous fistulae. The fluid can be more easily collected in a stoma bag although adhering the flange may be difficult as the fistula opening is usually flat and is rarely in a convenient place. Time needs to be spent finding the ideal appliance and tailoring its attachment to the fistula. If the opening is small and the output liquid, insertion of a urinary catheter may allow greater control and avoid skin contact. The balloon is gently inflated with the catheter placed inside the stoma bag.

Vesicovaginal fistulae

Continual leakage of urine causes soreness of the perineal skin. If the bladder is voided regularly this can help somewhat. Occasionally, insertion of a urinary catheter gives relief, but can be uncomfortable as it gives rise to bladder irritation and spasm. Using less fluid in the catheter balloon may reduce this.

The skin should be cleaned regularly and a barrier cream applied. Non-bulky absorbent pads may be of use. A tampon can absorb small leaks for short periods of time but may give unreliable control. In some cases, insertion of a nephrostomy tube or formation of an ileal conduit to divert urine flow has improved the quality of a patient's life.

Lymphoedema

Swelling of the lower limbs can occur in isolation or together with oedema of the trunk and genital area. The lymphatics may be damaged as a result of cancer, radiotherapy, or surgery. In progressive disease there is usually concomitant hypoalbuminaemia, immobility, and venous obstruction which will all exacerbate the condition. Deep-vein thrombosis can further complicate the issue.

Lymphoedema is best managed at an early stage. The four cornerstones of management are: (1) massage, (2) skin care, (3) support, and (4) movement (Badger and Twycross 1988). The skin should be protected by moisturizing it regularly and care should be given to avoid skin damage. If infection occurs, this should be treated rapidly with antibiotics. After more than one episode a prolonged course should be prescribed. Some patients require long-term prophylaxis.

In moderate or severe lymphoedema, the limb or genitalia can be uncomfortable due to pressure and skin tightness together with associated stiffness of the joints.

Discomfort and pain should be treated with appropriate analgesia. Occasionally, diuretics can reduce the tightness of the affected limb, although they rarely help with the swelling. High dose steroids may be beneficial, reducing tumour bulk and perivascular oedema. If a trial of steroids fails to be of benefit they should be stopped as, conversely, they may also aggravate swelling. Gentle massage of the trunk far away from the affected areas can improve lymphatic flow. Compression hosiery may be helpful but should be avoided if there is generalized lower body oedema where fluid is pushed from one place to another. If both legs are affected, tights may be better than stockings as they can give gentle pressure to the genitalia and lower abdomen. Compression bandaging over absorbent dressings may be effective where skin is broken and weeping (lymphorrhoea).

Fungating tumours

Fungating tumours commonly occur in vulval and cervical malignancy, but can also result from skin metastases or spread to a stoma site or a scar (laparotomy or from ascitic drainage). A fungating tumour is distressing because of the appearance and the odour from necrotic tissue. This can lead to social isolation and loss of intimacy within the family. Pain can be due to skin and muscle infiltration and may be aggravated by inflammation as a result of treatment or infection. In particular, pain may be a problem at the time of dressing changes which may need to be frequent to reduce odour.

Radiotherapy or surgery should be considered as treatment options in the management of fungating tumours. By controlling local disease both pain and smell can be improved. For skin soreness, topical local anaesthetic gels may be a useful short-term measure. Rapidly acting opioid drugs can be given 20–30 minutes prior to dressing changes if these are painful (immediate-release morphine or dextromoramide, Palfium). Alternatively, nitrous oxide and oxygen mixture (Entonox) can be used during the procedure.

Inflammation and pain due to infection may be helped by antibiotics. Extended courses should be avoided. Necrotic tissue is susceptible to microbial colonization and metronidazole gel, which reduces odour and colonization, does not treat overwhelming infection (Newman *et al.* 1989). Where there is capillary bleeding, this can be reduced by using adrenaline-soaked gauze while changing dressings. Tranexamic acid applied topically or given orally may also help with haemostasis. Many of the newer dressings such as the alginates are haemostatic. The dressing used should be absorbent to prevent maceration of surrounding skin and fibre-free to reduce infection and allow for ease of removal.

Renal failure secondary to ureteric obstruction

Uraemia secondary to ureteric obstruction is a common event in gynae-cological malignancy. Any intervention should be considered carefully, as a relatively peaceful death due to uraemia may be preferable to one due to bleeding or infection.

In rare instances, high dose steroids may have a temporary delaying effect on progressive uraemia, by reducing oedema associated with disease compressing the ureters. The more invasive percutaneous insertion of a nephrostomy is a widely available and fairly easily performed procedure. Complications of treatment include morbidity due to dislodged or blocked tubes and infections often requiring intravenous antibiotics. In patients with advanced disease, survival may be prolonged, but quality of life can be poor. Studies have shown that the time spent at home after the procedure can be relatively short (Feuer *et al.* 1991; Kehoe *et al.* 1993). Patient selection is very important. Women who may benefit from a nephrostomy are those who have a cancer which may be treated with radiotherapy or chemo-therapy (Soper *et al.* 1988). Most patients with renal failure due to progressive untreatable carcinoma are not suitable candidates.

As renal function deteriorates it is important to adjust medication to allow for reduced renal excretion of drugs and metabolites (e.g. morphine).

Anorexia and weight loss

Cachexia, a syndrome of anorexia and weight loss associated with cancer, is often multi-factorial in nature. Combined with a relative decline in food intake, hypophagia, the syndrome is characterized by a chronic abnormal metabolic state with changes in carbohydrate, fat, and protein metabolism. Decreased appetite is a frequent complaint and is often more of a concern to the family than for the patient.

Hypophagia may result from changes in taste and smell or chronic nausea due to treatment. The tumour itself can cause obstruction. Circulating tumour products and host cytokines probably also decrease appetite.

Nausea should be treated and the avoidance of the sight, sounds and smells of meal preparation, and the intake of small frequent meals, may be helpful. Dietary supplements can be used and may offer psychological benefit. Drugs that have been used to improve appetite are progestogens, corticosteroids, and artificial cannabinoids. Studies in patients with non-endocrine responsive cancer show that progestogens, such as megestrol acetate, improve appetite and food intake and have, in some cases, been shown to stimulate weight gain. Corticosteroids have been shown to improve appetite and well-being, but rarely result in weight gain. All of these drugs have side-effects that may not be tolerable for the patient.

Ascites

Ascites commonly presents as an uncomfortable distension of the abdomen together with bloating. Other symptoms can be anorexia, nausea (with or without vomiting), heartburn, and dyspnoea. The commonest cause in gynaecological malignancy is ovarian cancer where ascites is present in up to 30 percent of women at the time of diagnosis and up to 60 percent at the time of death. Chemotherapy aimed at the active treatment of ovarian cancer may control ascites, but at the later stages palliative measures are required. The use of diuretics, such as spironolactone with frusemide to initiate diuresis, may be effective but can result in significant dehydration and should be used with caution. Often, paracentesis is necessary to give relief of distension, pain, and dyspnoea. Diuretics may delay the re-formation of ascites after paracentesis but should be discontinued if they fail to help.

The use of peritoneovenous shunts in malignant ascites is only rarely of benefit. They tend to block easily as a result of the high protein content of ascitic fluid. There is also a significant peri-operative mortality and morbidity from sepsis and thromboembolism.

Dyspnoea

Dyspnoea may be due to cancer or to concominant disease such as infection or obstructive airways disease. Pleural effusions, lung metastases, and lymphangitis carcinomatosa are the most frequent direct causes, with pulmonary emboli a common indirect cause. Treatment of a specific problem can give great symptom relief (e.g. antibiotics, drainage of an effusion, and corticosteroids for lymphangitis).

Breathlessness, a very subjective symptom, is increasingly mentioned as a problem when patients deteriorate. In many cases a specific cause cannot be found and it may be attributed to generalized weakness and debility. Anxiety is frequently present which can make the feeling worse. The fear of being suffocated and of stopping breathing during the night are common and can make night-time a worry. Reassurance is often needed and simple things such as company, a night-light, or a fan can be helpful.

The general feeling of breathlessness can be improved by reducing anxiety and lowering the respiratory drive. Diazepam given in small doses (2–5 mg) morning and night, together with regular oral morphine may help to achieve this. Respiratory depression tends not to be a problem when the drugs are introduced in low doses and titrated up. Sudden attacks of breathlessness or panic attacks can be eased by sublingual lorazepam (0.5–1 mg) which acts rapidly. Morphine given by a nebulizer has been used and is currently being evaluated.

The dying patient

When a patient is dying it is important to stop all treatments, drugs, and investigations that are not necessary. Analgesia and anti-emetics should be continued. Analgesic requirements can increase at this time and it is important that this is reviewed regularly and that prescribing practice reflects this. If terminal agitation or restlessness occurs it is important to exclude simple causes such as pain, urinary retention, or faecal impaction. If there is renal impairment, accumulation of drugs may be an aggravating factor. Agitation is often due to the dying process. Medication such as midazolam (initially 20–30 mg over 24 hours) or methotrimeprazine (25–50 mg initially over 24 hours) are useful given subcutaneously by continuous infusion.

Chestiness due to retained secretions tend to cause the family and staff more distress than the patient. Parenteral fluids should be stopped and subcutaneous hyoscine may help to alleviate this problem.

Other terminal events should be anticipated. Even if an anti-emetic is not required regularly, one should be prescribed in case it is needed. If haemorrhage is a possibility, for example with a deep, ulcerating groin lesion, then midazolam or another rapidly acting anxiolytic should be prescribed.

If the patient has expressed a wish about where they would like to die efforts should be made to ensure that the request is fulfilled. However, it may not be possible or appropriate to move a sick person in their last days. In any event, the patient and their family have a right to peaceful and, if possible, private surroundings where she can die with dignity and respect.

References

Ashby, M. A., Game, P. A., Devitt, P. *et al.* (1991). Percutaneous gastrostomy as a venting procedure in palliative care. *Palliative Medicine*, 5, 147–50.

Badger, C. and Twycross, R. G. (1988). Management of lymphoedema—Guidelines. Sobell Study Centre, Oxford.

Baines, M., Oliver, D. J., and Carter, R. L. (1985). Medical management of intestinal obstruction in patients with advanced malignant disease. A clinical and pathological study. *Lancet*, ii, 990–3.

Bristow, A. and Foster, J. M. G. (1988). Lumbar sympathectomy in the management of rectal sympathetic pain. *Annals of the Royal College of Surgeons of England*, 70, 38–9.

Bruera, E., de Stoutz, N. D., Fasinger, R. L. *et al.* (1995). Comparison of two different concentrations of hyaluronidase in patients receiving one hour infusions of hypodermoclysis. *Journal of Pain and Symptom Management*, 10, 505–9.

Castell, D. O. (1985). Calcium channel blocking agents for gastrointestinal disorders. *American Journal of Cardiology*, 55, 210B–13B.

Ernst, E.S., MacDonald, R. M., Paterson, A. H. G. *et al.* (1992). A double blind crossover trial of IV clodronate in metastatic bone pain. *Journal of Pain and Symptom Management*, 7, 4–11.

Faisinger, R. L., MacEachern, T., Miller, M. J. *et al.* (1994). The use of hypodermoclysis for rehydration in terminally ill cancer patients. *Journal of Pain and Symptom Management*, 9, 298–302.

Feuer, G. A., Fruchter, R., Seruri, E. *et al.* (1991). Selection for percutaneous nephrostomy in gynecologic cancer patients. *Gynecologic Oncology*, 42, 60–3.

Hendrickx, P., Orth, G., and Grunert, J. H. (1995). Long-term survival after embolisation of potentially lethal bleeding malignant pelvic tumours. *British Journal of Radiology*, 68, 1336–43.

IASP (International Association for the Study of Pain) (1986). Subcommittee on taxonomy classification of chronic pain. *Pain* (Suppl. 3), 216–21.

Kehoe, S., Luesley, D. M., Budden, J., and Earl, H. (1993). Percutaneous nephrostomies in woman with cervical cancer. *British Journal of Obstetrics and Gynaecolgy*, 100, 283–8.

MacGregor, K. J., Ahmedzai, S., Riley, J. *et al.* (1994). Symptomatic relief of excoriating skin conditions using a topical themoreversible gel. *Palliative Medicine*, 8, 76–7.

Mercadante, S., Spoldi, E., Caraceni, A. *et al.* (1993). Octreotide in relieving gastrointestinal symptoms due to bowel obstruction. *Palliative Medicine*, 7, 295–9.

Newman, V., Allwood, M., and Oakes, R. A. (1989). The use of metronidazole gel to control the smell of malodourous lesions. *Palliative Medicine*, 3, 303–5.

Nubiola-Calonge, P., Badia, J. M., Sancho, J. *et al.* (1987). Blind evaluation of the effect of octreotide, a somatostatin analogue, on small bowel fistula output. *Lancet*, ii, 672–3.

Portenoy, R. K. (1993). Adjuvant analgesics in pain management. In *Oxford textbook of palliative medicine* (ed. D. Doyle, G. W. C. Hanks, and N. MacDonald), Chapter 4, pp. 187–203.

Soper, J. T., Blaszczyk, T. M., Oke, E. *et al.* (1988). Percutaneous nephrostomy in gynecologic oncology patients. *American Journal of Obstetrics and Gynecology*, 5, 1126–31.

Twycross, R. (1994). *Pain relief in advanced cancer*, pp. 263–6. Churchill Livingstone, Edinburgh.

WHO (World Health Organization) (1986). *Cancer pain relief*. WHO, Geneva.

WHO (World Health Organization) (1990). Cancer pain relief and palliative care. *Technical report series 804*. WHO, Geneva.

Index

ablation 61, 115, 158
accelerated hyperfractionation 175–6
actinomycin-D 39, 214–15
adenoacanthomas 79
adenocarcinomas 4, 131
  of cervix 47, 51, 59–60, 70–1, 144, 164
    in situ (ACIS) 70, 71
    invasive 70–1
  clear cell 17–18, 71, 79, 82, 85, 86, 112, 118
  endometrial 79, 82, 85, 86, 88, 164
  endometrioid 17, 18, 77, 79, 95
  mucinous 17, 21
  of ovary 12, 17–18, 21, 34, 41
  serous 12, 17, 41, 79, 82, 85, 86
  of vagina 112, 114, 118
  of vulva 100, 101, 111
adenoid cystic tumours
  of Bartholin's glands 111
  cervical 71
adenosarcomas 95
adenosquamous carcinomas 70–1, 79, 82
alkylating agents 29–31, 209–13, 218, 222, 228, 233
  see also named drugs
alopecia 31, 212, 213, 216, 218, 227–8
alpha:beta ratio 174, 175
alpha fetoprotein (FP) 22, 36, 38, 39
anaemia 225
analgesics 238–45, 255
anaphylactic shock 223
anaplastic tumours 5
androgens, aromatization of 76
aneuploid tumours 34–5, 86, 141, 142, 145
angiogenesis 35, 70

anorexia and weight loss 254
anthracyclines 92, 94, 95, 208, 213–14, 227, 228, 230, 232–3
  see also named drugs
antibiotics 158, 225, 250, 252, 253
  cytotoxic 29, 213–15; *see also named drugs*
anticonvulsants 244, 245
antidepressants 243–4
anti-emetics 226, 241, 246, 248, 255
antimetabolites 29, 32, 215–16, 232
  see also named drugs
apoptosis 138, 139, 234
ascites 90, 215, 226, 254
  and ovarian cancer 19, 20, 21, 24, 25, 26

Bartholin's glands 99
  carcinomas of 101, 111
basal cell carcinomas 110
B cell lymphomas 141
BCG (Bacille Calmette–Guérin) 34
becquerels (Bq) 177
Bethesda System 51
bidigital examination 156
bimanual examination 56, 156
biological agents in cervical cancer 69–70
biologically equivalent doses 175
bladder, radiation damage to 201–2
bladder drainage 163
bladder dysfunction after surgery 168
bladder mucosa, bullous oedema of 57
bladder reference point 194
bleomycin 39, 69, 109, 214, 219, 223, 225, 230
blood count monitoring 225